DIVINE NOURISHMENT FOR
SELF-LOVE AND RADIANT HEALTH

THE
SECRET
OF
FOOD

CAROLIN EICKHOFF

The Secret of Food:
Divine Nourishment for Self-Love and Radiant Health

carolineickhoff.com

Published by Made to Change the World™ Publishing
Nashville, Tennessee

Cover and interior design by Chelsea Jewell

Paperback ISBN: 978-1-956837-35-3
Ebook ISBN: 978-1-956837-36-0

Printed in the USA, Canada, Australia, and Europe

To you, the brave soul dedicated to nourishing yourself physically, emotionally, and spiritually.

I *see* you.

I *celebrate* you.

May you find within these words the wisdom to free yourself from guilt and restriction and nourish your body with kindness and compassion.

You've got this!

CONTENTS

CHAPTER 6

EASE & GRACE

page 75

CHAPTER 7

TRUTH & TRUST

page 87

LOVE FOOD RECIPES

page 95

ACKNOWLEDGMENTS

This book would not have been possible without the love, support, and guidance of numerous individuals who have played pivotal roles in shaping both my personal journey and the message conveyed within these pages.

First and foremost, I am profoundly grateful to my family for their enduring love and encouragement throughout every step of my journey. Their unwavering belief in me has been my greatest source of strength.

To my mentor and friend Britnie Turner—through your example, you gave me the strength to create my organization, which produces the Love Ball gourmet chocolate in a climate-friendly and sustainable manner and also supports social projects for children in Tanzania. Thank you for your dedication to humanity and Aerial Recovery's mission to save lives and stop evil. Your commitment to creating positive change in the world serves as a beacon of hope, reminding me of the profound impact that one individual can make. Your vision and leadership exemplify the transformative power of compassion and action, inspiring me to strive for excellence in all my endeavors.

To Brooke and Brett Thomas, your support and friendship have been a constant source of encouragement and inspiration. Amare=love. Your belief and faith in my vision and dedication to my success have fueled my determination to make a positive impact in the world.

To Peta Kelly, your fearless approach to entrepreneurship and commitment to living a purpose-driven life have inspired me to embrace my authenticity and pursue my passions with fierce determination. Your empowering message of abundance and self-love continues to resonate deeply with me, reminding me to live each day with intention and gratitude.

Thank you to Jamie Kern Lima. Your trailblazing spirit in the beauty industry has left an indelible mark. Your journey from struggling entrepreneur to founder of a billion-dollar cosmetics empire is a testament to perseverance and resilience. Your commitment to inclusivity and authenticity has redefined standards of beauty, inspiring millions to embrace their uniqueness. Thank you for your courage, innovation, and relentless pursuit of empowering others to feel confident in their own skin.

To Tony Robbins, your unparalleled expertise in the field of personal development has been a constant source of inspiration. Your teachings have not only enriched my own life but have also profoundly influenced the message I seek to share with others through this book.

Endless gratitude to Jamie Oliver, a disruptor in the food industry, whose innovative approach to culinary excellence

ACKNOWLEDGMENTS

has forever changed the way I perceive nourishment. Your dedication to promoting sustainable food practices has inspired me to adopt a more conscious approach to eating and living.

To Willie Harcourt-Cooze, your pioneering work in the chocolate industry has not only delighted the taste buds of millions but has also served as a catalyst for positive change. Your commitment to ethical sourcing and environmental sustainability sets a shining example for all.

Deep appreciation to Dr. Bob Murray, whose groundbreaking contributions to the world of sports nutrition have revolutionized the way athletes fuel their bodies. Your dedication to optimizing performance through wholesome, nutrient-rich foods has had a profound impact on the lives of countless individuals.

To Oprah Winfrey, your tireless advocacy for health and wellness has made a lasting impression on me and countless others. Your passion for empowering individuals to take control of their health and live their best lives is truly inspiring.

Heartfelt thanks to Eckhart Tolle, a luminary in the field of mindfulness and self-discovery. Your teachings on cultivating inner peace and embracing the present moment have profoundly influenced my own journey of self-discovery and personal growth.

To Vandana Shiva, your innovative contributions to the field of sustainable agriculture have paved the way for a more resilient and equitable food system. Your commitment to environmental stewardship and social responsibility serves as a beacon of hope for future generations.

Thank you, Mark Zuckerberg, for your revolutionary impact on communication and connectivity through Facebook, which allows me to share my message with a global audience.

To Roger Federer, your grace and excellence on the tennis court inspire me to pursue greatness with humility and determination.

Teal Swan, your discerning insights into spirituality and personal growth have deepened my understanding of self-discovery and inner healing. I am forever changed.

Deep gratitude to Gabriela Gastberg for her dedication to empowering me every day. You are simply the best! I am so thankful for the life we live together. Thank you for believing in me and making it possible for all the people on this Earth to find true happiness. The Best!

To the British Royal Family, your dedication to philanthropy and public service sets a shining example. May everyone contribute on such a level.

Tobias Beck, your thoughtful insights into personal development and entrepreneurship have been a guiding light on my journey. Your teachings have challenged and motivated me to push beyond my limits, embracing discomfort as a catalyst for growth. Thank you for your wisdom, guidance, and unwavering belief in the power of transformation.

ACKNOWLEDGMENTS

Peter Tabichi, your selfless dedication to education and uplifting impoverished communities in Kenya serves as a beacon of hope and inspiration to all.

Les Brown, thank you for your wisdom, inspiration, and transformative teachings. Through them, you have guided me on my path to personal growth and self-discovery.

Brené Brown, your research on vulnerability has shaped the way I view courage and inspired me to embrace authenticity. Thank you for demonstrating the power of owning your story.

Jack Canfield, your teachings have been a beacon of light for me on the path to personal growth. Your timeless wisdom and practical strategies have empowered me and millions of others to unlock their potential and achieve their dreams.

To Her Royal Highness Princess Reema, your visionary leadership and commitment to empowering women and youth in Saudi Arabia exemplify the power of compassion and inclusivity in society.

Rihanna, your fearless creativity and commitment to social justice have sparked important conversations and driven meaningful change.

P!nk, your raw honesty and empowering lyrics have uplifted countless souls, including mine, reminding me to embrace my uniqueness and stand up for what I believe in.

Tina Turner, your resilience and passion for music remind me to channel my own inner strength and creativity in pursuing my dreams.

To the Cardone family, your dedication to entrepreneurship and philanthropy serves as a testament to the power of hard work, determination, and generosity in shaping a better world for all. Thank you for your example.

Thank you, Dr. Deepak Chopra, for your wisdom and insight. They have been instrumental in shaping my perspective on holistic wellness and sustainable nutrition. Your guidance has been invaluable.

And last, but certainly not least, my deepest heartfelt gratitude to those on a courageous journey of self-love and self-acceptance, especially in a world that often demands conformity to unrealistic standards. I honor each of you who dares to challenge societal norms and expectations, embracing your bodies and defying societal pressures to change. Radical self-love is your war cry and your efforts are not in vain; they are seeds of change that will cultivate a more compassionate and inclusive world. Love fully and shine brightly!

FOREWORD

Too often, people receive the message that they are unworthy—unworthy of success, unworthy of beauty, unworthy of health, unworthy of love, unworthy of living a remarkable life by living out loud.

Carolin Eickhoff received that message ... even from herself. Especially from herself. Like so many others, Carolin had a toxic relationship with food. For most of her life, her weight and eating habits resulted in poor health. And she was given the message over and over that her problematic relationship with food was simply her fate based on her family history ... her genes ... the literal way she was built. She internalized that message to the point where she actually sabotaged herself every time she thought about getting healthy. Why bother trying—she wasn't worthy!

How often have you heard that same message? Whether it's about your body, your mind, or your soul, you've probably told yourself, at some point, that you're not worth it. While Carolin's journey is specifically about weight loss and health, anyone reading this book can certainly extrapolate the bigger message of self-acceptance and self-love. It's about reclaiming one's worth, embracing one's true identity, and walking boldly in the purpose for which we were created. It's about learning to love oneself—body, mind, and soul—and extending that love to others in a world desperately in need of compassion and grace.

In *The Secret of Food: Divine Nourishment for Self-Love and Radiant Health*, Carolin tells the story about changing not only a body that limited her, that kept her from living a life she desired, but, more importantly, about changing her view of herself to one of love. And Carolin knows of what she speaks.

I met Carolin years ago. After she attended one of my in-person events, I learned about the Love Ball—her good-for-you, good-for-the-Earth, and good-for-the-world nourishing gourmet chocolates that are produced through sustainable, organic, and fair trade principles. Since then, our friendship has deepened as I've watched her develop and expand her mission to coach people to overcome toxic relationships with food and regain their health.

Since 2016, through her My Best Version Academy, and, more recently, her My Best Version podcast, she's been guiding others to sustainably achieve a body that they love to live in—one that is healthy, feels good, and enables them to live their best lives. She helps her clients overcome yo-yo cravings; select, prepare, and enjoy food that results in long-term sustainable weight loss; reframe their body perception and body image; and, ultimately, achieve transformations of body, mind, and soul!

Carolin's story is one of resilience, redemption, and unwavering faith. From the depths of despair, she has risen, shedding not only pounds but also the shackles of self-doubt and insecurity.

Her transformation is nothing short of miraculous, a testament to the power of belief and the resilience of the human spirit.

And it reminds me of the profound truth that we are fearfully and wonderfully made, each of us a masterpiece in the hands of a loving Creator. No matter how far we may stray or how broken we may feel, there is always hope for redemption and restoration. Carolin's story is an example that we are capable of far more than we can imagine when we surrender to the guiding hand of divine grace.

As you embark on this journey through Carolin's story, may you be inspired to live out loud—to embrace your true identity, to pursue your passions with boldness and conviction, and to extend love and grace to yourself and others in every moment.

With love and gratitude,
Brooke Thomas

INTRODUCTION

My body limited me for years, which meant I didn't live the life I really wanted. It felt like my insides didn't match my outsides. My life was characterized by behavior that was harmful to my health and my body and contributed to me developing type 2 diabetes at the age of 18 and weighing 265 pounds (120 kilograms). I needed change, but my attempts were short-lived and unsustainable. I heard from my family, my doctors, and myself that it was useless to even try … that I should just accept my body and the limitations it caused.

Life was so loud, full of so many people's voices, so many inputs, and so many voices in my own head that all I knew with any degree of certainty was that I needed to get away. I needed a change of scenery to be alone with my own crappy thoughts.

For me, that meant getting out into nature where I could be in stillness and quiet—away from routines, away from any distractions, away from busyness, away from all the opinions of others. The outside noise felt like a giant boombox that was about to explode. I needed a real break. I needed myself again.

And so I went on a journey into nature, and there began my first cycle of losing the weight.

But despite initially losing the exterior weight at that time, I didn't free myself from the interior weight. I wasn't dealing with the real emotions, the root causes underneath all the layers.

I wasn't able to look at myself in the mirror and be honest about what I was thinking and feeling and how I got where I was. Even without the distractions, even without the noise, I still wasn't able to hear the truth about myself. I needed to get quiet, really quiet, and intimate with myself. I needed to find out exactly what I was avoiding. But the stillness and quiet only turned the volume up on those voices in my head, and all I could hear was hatred for myself ... blame ... shame ... guilt. I had tried to change my body from a place of anger and frustration, not from a place of love.

After this time alone, even after losing the exterior weight, I felt worse than ever before. I was still disgusted with my body, with myself. I was doing everything that I thought would solve the problem, everything that I thought would ease the pain, everything that I thought would heal the trauma. I did everything that *they* said I should do to magically be happy. But I wasn't happy. I wasn't healed. I wasn't kind to myself. And I didn't show myself grace.

I felt so empty and alone despite doing everything I was told would make me feel whole. And then I hated myself even more because I had put myself through such torture for nothing. The same misery, the same emptiness, the same loneliness, the same rage, the same pain. Only now my knees and my back hurt. I was hungry all the time. My muscles were sore. Hell, I couldn't even sit on the toilet. The restrictions I put on myself through food and exercise worked physically, but only for a while. Eventually, even the exterior weight came back.

For years, I had thought that reaching that point, the point where I had lost all the weight and would fit into a fantastic dress, would make me happy. That I would be able to finally love myself and be proud of myself. Instead, I sat on the floor of my bedroom in front of the scale, weighing the "perfect" weight, tears streaming down my face, miserable. How did I get here? Why did I feel worse than ever before? How was that possible?

I may have reached a point on my scale that felt lighter, but I was very heavy inside. Suddenly, I heard my inner voice loud and clear: "I told you to be soft because I need you to be kind to us." All the effort, the extreme workouts, starving myself, going to bed at 5:00 p.m. because I had no energy left was self-punishment. It was at that moment that I realized there had to be another way. I had a vision of myself living as a woman in peace and freedom, someone who was able to breathe physically and emotionally.

I had an intense urge to scream out loud. And you know what? That's what I did. I took off my dress, put on my running shoes, and walked down the street. I started running, screaming, and shouting from the top of my lungs. People were staring at me, wondering what was happening to me. But I didn't care. I was tired of being the good girl, doing all the right things, trying to fix everything. I was exhausted from trying to do what I had been told to do. Every perfection that I sought on the outside left me lonely and in an even darker place on the inside than I was before. After jumping, screaming, punching my fists in the air, clapping, and stamping on the ground, I felt incredibly free. I started talking out loud to myself. "Yes, this is what we are going to do, Carolin. Yes, we did it once, and we are doing it again because we are here and we are meant to live a life that is worth living. To experience a life where we feel good on the inside and shine that light on the outside, that's why we are here. That's why we are here."

I noticed a shift in my awareness. I started cheering myself on instead of pushing myself down. I started talking to my body as *we*, a communion, a team.

I knew there had to be a way to feel better about myself and to be happier because other people were doing it. And so I began to search to discover why some people could lose the weight, could find the joy, could be in the relationship, could be happy, could walk in their purpose, could be fulfilled—and why others, like me, couldn't.

Self-love took on an entirely different meaning. A deeper meaning. I hadn't known that it actually existed, that it was more than just an intellectual exercise. I started to understand what true self-love feels, smells, tastes, sounds, and looks like. It felt like golden nectar that I could sense all around me, a sweet honey that was pouring into all of the cracks in my life, and I became curious to know how I could embody this sweetness. So I set out to discover the secret, and I found it. This book is in honor of what I found. For now, I will tell you that there is a happy ending. When I uncovered the secret, I lost the weight, gained the joy, found peace within myself, and met the man of my dreams. My hope is that this book will help you find your happy ending, too.

So this book is written from my heart to yours. I see you, I feel you, I relate to you because I am you. Whenever you feel down, stuck, or you're questioning yourself, I want you to come back to this book and read through these lines again. I've poured my heart into this book to remind you of who you truly are. You're worthy of and meant to live a life full of laughter, fun, and passion. I want you to feel yummy in all the areas of your life because this is how you have been designed to live.

It's time for you to unlock and unleash your superpowers to be a greater force for good in this world. It's your time now to shine. It's time for you to express yourself in your unique way. There is no one more capable of living your life than you.

CHAPTER 1
REAL TALK

Let's Get Real

There was a time in my life when I weighed 265 pounds (120 kilograms). I was diabetic, sick, lonely, and miserable; every day felt painful, and I felt so hopeless.

Maybe you're there, too.

But your journey to self-love begins today. Your journey to happiness starts now. Your journey to freedom and joy and a lifetime of who you truly are is yours for the taking. But, in order for you to take that journey, it's important for you to be real with yourself.

Take a few moments to contemplate the following questions:
- Do you feel empty?
- Are you trying to escape pain?
- Are you hiding from something?
- Are you trying to forget an event or circumstance from the past?
- What brought you here?

Be honest so that you can create the path forward. Whatever your responses, those were moments in time, a season of your life. You are not broken. There is a reason you have not given up. This is not your fate.

Now is a new moment, and here begins a new season.
- So what do you long for?
- What do you want?
- How would you like to feel?

Give yourself permission to dream.
- How active would you like to be?
- How would you like to play with your children or your grandchildren?
- What adventures would you like to go on?
- What relationships would you like to have?

These are the questions to ask yourself to develop a vision of what you want your life to look like.

To help you navigate this process, I've created prompts and a worksheet that you can download from my website at carolineeickhoff.com/free. I encourage you to take a few minutes for yourself and really be honest about what's going on in your life, how you got here, and where you want to go. Because it's that clarity, that vision, that's going to be the fuel that propels you through this journey.

It's a journey of reconnecting with yourself, of loving yourself, of shining your light, of showing up fully as you—for your family, for your friends, for your community, for your world, and, most importantly, for yourself.

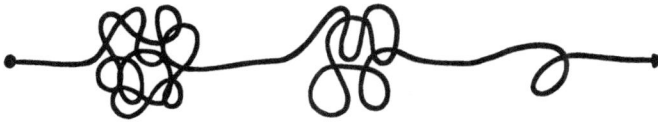

The Moment of Decision

You're fed up. You've reached the point of "no more" … not another minute, another hour, another day. You feel overwhelmed and undervalued. Maybe you haven't yet reached the tipping point, but you know that something is different. *Maybe* you're starting to understand that changing your life is as simple as the next decision you make.

It is in the moments of decision that your destiny is shaped. So whether you've been at that tipping point before or you're at a crossroads right now, the first step toward freedom and self-love is *deciding* that you want to take the journey … *deciding* that you're worth the exploration … *deciding* that you want the outcome you desire.

These moments when your entire life makes a U-turn can be very painful because you know that your life will never be the same again. But they also have the potential to be the best moments! Change is hard, and being fully alive in the painful moments is hard, but it can be done.

There was a moment where I knew I had to change today—not yesterday and not next week. It was the turning point in my life. In 2013, I got a phone call from my doctor. She informed me that my blood results weren't good, and I needed to come in as soon as possible. I knew exactly what was going on; her phone call confirmed that my relationship with food was making me sick … that I was living in a state of illness from the weight. I also knew that I had been playing small my whole life. I had been hiding—hiding behind dark clothes, hiding my voice, hiding who I was, and I was hurting myself. At that moment, I was overcome by a sense of urgency. I … had … to … change. That was the point in my journey when I started moving away from the noise and spending even more time in nature. With that one phone call, I knew all of this, and I had reached a breaking point where I knew I had the choice to step up and choose myself and my life or give up. In that moment, I decided to take ownership of my health and take responsibility for my body, my weight, and, especially, my happiness.

I remember that it was pouring rain, and yet, from somewhere within me, I heard a voice asking me to go outside and run. This moment couldn't have been a more perfect moment for change. I stopped trying to find the best way, the best timing, the best sequence of events for when I was supposed to change. I just did it. I didn't have any trainers, no sports leggings. I just went outside and ran. In the pouring rain, in my slippers, my own voice in my head screaming at me, yelling at me, laughing at me to go back inside, to stay comfortable. But my heart knew that in that moment when I chose to run, it would be the moment that changed my life. It was the moment, the one decision, that shifted the trajectory of my life and my health forever.

The Moment of No Return

You know the saying the journey of a thousand miles starts with the first step? It really does. I was so afraid of change. I was so overwhelmed with all the emotions, trying to make the process perfect, to take the perfect actions, to be obedient, to make sure I changed my life in the perfect way. I wanted to control everything. I wanted to see all the way to the end. I wanted to know where I was going and how I was going to get there. But I realized that I needed to focus on one step at a time. And that's what I did. One step at a time, one run at a time. I felt good after taking the first step because it was a feeling of stepping up for myself as well as a literal first step; even if nobody was there cheering me on, even if nobody was there to say that I was doing well, I did it for myself. I made the decision and declaration for me and my heart as an act of prioritizing myself. That was one of the best moments of my life. My heart smiled because there was a part of me that knew that I *could* have it all by taking one step, and then taking that one step again and again, consistently and in a self-loving way, without judgment and shame. I had never known how to love myself. I didn't know how it felt to have love for myself. I didn't know I should make decisions from a place of love, but I was starting to become curious about it all. I said to myself, "Well, what you've done up until now hasn't worked, so let's find out what happens if you try doing it from love instead of from hate." This was the point of no return.

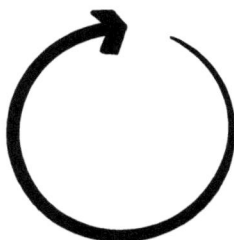

There was a quest that had been placed in my heart to experience my life to the fullest, and I knew I had to listen to the call. All these dreams had been placed in my heart by God to live out loud and in my reality, not just in my imagination. If it wasn't possible to live them, I wouldn't have the amazing dreams in the first place. I anchored this moment of stepping up for myself with a song that would allow me to stay in the flow I had during these realizations. This song enables me to harness the energy I felt in those moments whenever I need to channel it.

I invite you to spend a few minutes finding a song that energizes you and reminds you of self-love. It must be a song that gives you a good feeling and sets you in motion. A song you can listen to over and over again when life gets tough, when life is easy, when you want to celebrate, or when you want to honor yourself. This song will become your war cry, so find a song that makes you feel alive.

Walk the Walk

One of the biggest lessons I had to learn along my journey was walking the walk. I had to learn to dance my way through the ups and downs, the mountains and valleys of life. Life happens. You are a beautiful soul in a human body, and you are here to experience all of life, in all of its glorious unpredictability. Walking the walk means being able to have lasting joy and happiness—happiness that is not dependent on external factors. This was key to my self-discovery journey. I didn't want another quick fix or another pushup. I wanted to experience true, long-term, sustainable self-love, love from others, happiness, and health. After all, I couldn't serve others if I didn't go first. I had always been good at pleasing people, at suppressing my truth, fitting in, being in the background, supporting other people. But when it came to prioritizing myself, putting me in the front row, speaking up for myself, standing up for myself, and owning my truth, I had never been capable of doing any of it.

So there I was, open and ready to learn how to do just that. I remember sitting in a restaurant a couple of days after I had made the big decision to live from love. I pulled out my journal, opened it, and wrote on the top line of the left page: "What would a person who loves themselves do right now?" I was willing to change the story of my life to a story of love. I wanted my life to tell a story of play and fun and love for myself. But who was this person I was talking about? "Who am I?" I asked myself in the pages of my journal. I only knew that I was hiding—hiding in a body that wasn't me because I felt heavy in every way. I always had a big smile on my face, and people liked what I projected on the outside. Everybody thought I was happy. But on the inside, I was so unfulfilled. I was missing out on so much of the beauty of my life. During this moment, I became aware of a part of me inside my heart that wanted to come out. There was a little girl inside me that wasn't showing up on the outside. I asked myself, "How would it feel if my inside matched my outside? How would it feel to be a woman who is fulfilled on the inside and shining on the outside?" I desperately wanted both of these parts of myself to merge because I felt disconnected from who I really was. So I went from talking the talk to walking the walk. I had spent too much time in my head, thinking about what to do next, waiting to find the perfect answers. It was time to do something new. All beautiful beginnings start with beautiful new questions that lead in the direction of true happiness.

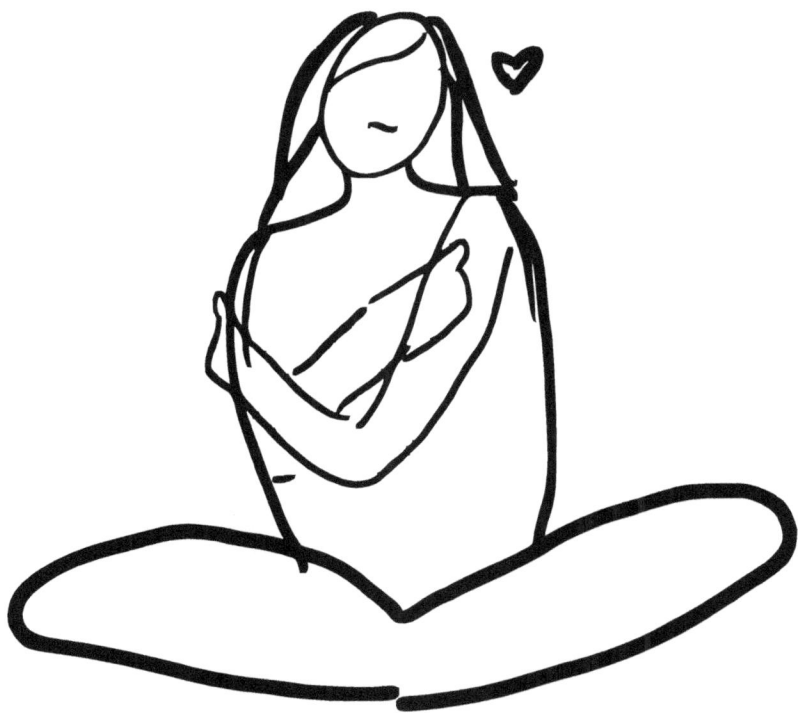

CHAPTER 2

SENSES

Intimacy and connection with myself and my body was the first step on my journey. When I first started walking this road, I didn't realize how disconnected I was from my body because I was numbing myself with distraction, overeating, and self-punishment—everything I could to avoid pain and my emotions. But I came to realize that if I numbed my negative emotions, then I would also numb my positive ones, like joy and happiness and love. And because I was looking for and wanting to experience what it meant to feel radiant love on the inside, I had to find a way back to union with myself and activate all of my senses and *all* of my emotions.

You can only truly experience love through your senses. Love isn't an intellectual process. It isn't logical. Love becomes fully alive when it is activated through your senses. And once you activate love, you will activate your potential. When you slow down and become more present in your life, in the midst of all the busyness, you will have a more profound relationship with your senses and be better able to explore them. This will enhance your ability to experience a range of emotions, allowing you to reconnect with the forgotten parts of yourself that have been lost underneath all the shame and insecurity. Love needs to be felt in the present moment so that you can accept God's truth as your reality: That you are love and you are loved.

Your senses are the route for your body to receive, experience, and express all the information from the world around you. They allow you to bask in the richness of life's bounty.

See

Sight is the tool used for seeing yourself and your divinity in all its different forms and variations. There is a difference between outwardly seeing yourself and recognizing who you are on a deeper level … one where you understand the inherent connection between everything around you and within you. There are no coincidences. Have you ever noticed that a walnut looks like your brain and is actually good for concentration? Or that a carrot, which is good for your sight, sliced in half looks like an eye? Between life, God, food, nature, and your body, everything is deeply connected and intertwined. When you eliminate all the distractions that you use in your everyday life, like addictions—to food, to people, to escape—your sight can open up. You will have new opportunities to be present in your body in a healthy way and notice energy, its connections and flow.

Look at your hands. Place them right in front of you and look at each of your fingers. Can you see all the beautiful fine lines and shapes that are patterned across your skin? Take a moment to become present to the hands that have carried you through this life. How do your fingers look? Can you see that your hands are shaped like the leaves of a tree? There is sacred geometry in your being, a beautiful way for you to become present to your life and your aliveness. This practice of taking time to see will ultimately lead to less stress from fast-paced modern life, especially within your body. This is one of the most crucial aspects of your journey—to find a way to become more present to your life, the world around you, the connections, and the energy. Notice how these practices regulate your nervous system. Notice how your nervous system exhales when you release yourself to the flow. For more practices, visit **carolineickhoff.com/free**.

Smell

Once, when I sat next to the ocean on a beautiful summer's day, I could feel the warm sand beneath my legs and feet. I took a deep breath in, and I noticed how much I loved the feeling of the ocean playing with my whole body. I loved the smell of the ocean. The salty breeze in the air made me feel alive. With every breath I took, I focused even more on the smells around me. I had a mango, my favorite fruit, in my hand, and I looked at it. "How beautiful are you," I said to the fruit. I was suddenly aware of an altered state of consciousness, and I heard an inner

THE SECRET OF FOOD

voice talking to me. "Smell. Smell my beautiful gift." I was taken
aback. The mango was talking to me! That was something I'd
never experienced before. "Yes, you're right, you can hear me.
Please smell me. I'm here for you to experience how fantastic
fruit can smell and what it does for your body." I was holding my
breath, realizing that I was sitting on the beach connecting with
the ocean, having a conversation with my mango. I thought,
"Yes, this is the life that I desire to live, a life where I am in
connection with everything in and around me."

If you are willing to make yourself uncomfortable, you will
discover extraordinary things. If you are always looking for love,
for God's love, in a certain form, you will miss the other ways
God shows up. Your sense of smell can bring you back to your
center, to connection, to the present and all of its magic.

Here is an exercise to help bring your awareness to smells. The
next time you see a rose, or any beautiful flower, don't just pass
by it. Touch her, smell her, connect with the beautiful incense of
her petals and her spirit of nature. Divine essence is all around,
inviting you to receive the medicine of smell.

Taste

Let's go back to the beautiful moment in the restaurant. After
I had finished writing in my journal about living from love, I
ordered one of my favorite dishes, and out came the fluffiest
pancakes I've ever tasted in my life. On top of my pancakes
were berries in all different colors. Raspberries, blueberries,
strawberries. I was fascinated. After allowing my senses to open

up more and more, I could see food in a completely different way … in a more wholesome way … in a way that nourished me … in a way that would enhance my beauty and my vitality. I then deeply understood that certain foods would rejuvenate me. While I sat in front of my plate staring at the beautiful berries that had been lovingly placed on my pancakes, I got the idea to eat them in a way that I'd never done with food before. I thought, "How would it taste if I close my eyes and use all my senses to enjoy my food in a sensual way?" I put on a smile, got my fork, and ate a piece of pancake.

It felt like I was eating a lover. The combination of sweet and sour and savory with eyes closed, being entirely present in my body, made me feel happy. For the first time in years, I enjoyed my food. I enjoyed eating the pancakes without any guilt, without any restrictions on how and what I should eat, or how much I should eat, or what my diet plan dictated, or any restrictions on colors or how many points were in the meal. I became free. I was free of all the diets, ideas, and trends in my mind. Thoughts of judgment came, but I could actually differentiate these thoughts from truth. I could observe them rather than *be* them.

I said to myself, "Stop." I wanted to enjoy my pancakes and berries without any thoughts clouding the experience. It was the first time in my life that I would consciously shut off my mind and choose a different way of thinking. My taste buds felt as if they were exploding into different universes because I could enjoy not only my food, but also myself enjoying my food. This was a very intimate experience for me. I could taste the colors. I could taste the flavors. I could taste the emotions in the food.

THE SECRET OF FOOD

I could taste the intensity of every bite, and I thought to myself, "Wow, this is what I need." At that moment, I was learning to love myself and eat in a way that was good for me. I opened myself up to experience pleasure in something as fundamental as feeding myself, nourishing myself. I was *tasting* food, maybe for the first time, instead of just filling my stomach. I tasted flavors I never knew existed. The taste of love was born.

Soon after, I found myself standing in my kitchen surrendering to the moment of now. I had no idea how to cook or even what to cook to recreate the feeling of love I had felt with the pancakes. I only knew I loved being present with myself. It felt so good to finally be listening to my body and talking to my food, like I was communicating with the Holy Spirit. It was wild. So intimate, so divine. I wanted more of those moments. This is how the Love Ball was born.

I started with what I had. I put together raw cacao nibs, dates, and raspberries. It tasted like love. I rolled it in my hands until it formed a ball, and God said, "It is done, it is here, it is born. Love is here right now. It's a Love Ball. Look at the beautiful creation you just made. You are a Love Ball. I made you, you are so loved." I started crying. I didn't know what had just happened, but I believed it. I felt a love like no other, maybe for the first time. I looked at the creation in my hands.

"Love Ball," He said. "This is the secret. I'm revealing my secret now to you. Use this ball as an act of love, with love, and in a way that shows others how I love. You are my most amazing daughter. I love you, and I want you to use this Love Ball and share this love I have for you. It's for all people, all humans on this planet, to be reminded of me, of God. People are suffering and hurting. I'm going to speak to them through the food to touch their hearts. Thank you for birthing this creation. I'm going to put you in spaces where people need me, where people need the Love Ball. Thank you for listening. This feeling you are feeling is the feeling of being nurtured. This is the taste of the divine."

The Love Ball began with cacao, dates, and raspberries, but it will soon grow into an entire divine nutrition collection with seven different varieties; each and every one will heal people and stop evil. The Love Ball heals the body-mind connection. This is food for purpose. Enjoy it, and let your body be a vessel and a clear channel for love.

The Love Ball chocolate reflects God's goodness in several ways by embodying His principles of love:

1. *Quality Ingredients:* Using high-quality ingredients sourced ethically and sustainably demonstrates a commitment to stewarding God's creation with care and respect. This reflects God's goodness in providing abundant resources for enjoyment and sustenance.

2. *Promoting Fairness and Equity:* Ensuring fair wages and working conditions for those involved in the production process reflects God's heart for justice and compassion. By treating all workers with dignity and respect, the Love Ball chocolate business exemplifies God's love for every individual.

3. *Bringing Joy and Celebration:* The act of enjoying chocolate can be a simple pleasure that brings happiness

and celebration. God delights in His people finding joy in His creation and experiencing His goodness.

4. *Supporting Community and Collaboration:* Partnering with local communities and organizations to promote social good and address pressing needs reflects God's desire for unity and collaboration among His people. The Love Ball chocolate business contributes to building stronger, more connected communities through its partnerships and initiatives.

5. *Giving Back and Making a Difference:* Allocating a portion of proceeds to charitable causes and community development projects demonstrates a commitment to serving others and making a positive impact. By supporting initiatives that align with God's heart for compassion and justice, the Love Ball chocolate business reflects His goodness and brings hope to those in need.

The Love Ball chocolate is a tangible expression of God's goodness and love in the world by embodying His principles of love, justice, compassion, and generosity. Through its practices, partnerships, and impact, the business is contributing to creating a more loving, equitable, and flourishing world, reflecting God's goodness to all.

By purchasing the Love Ball chocolate, you heal yourself and help save lives. Purchase a Love Ball here:

carolineickhoff.com/loveball

LOVE BALL

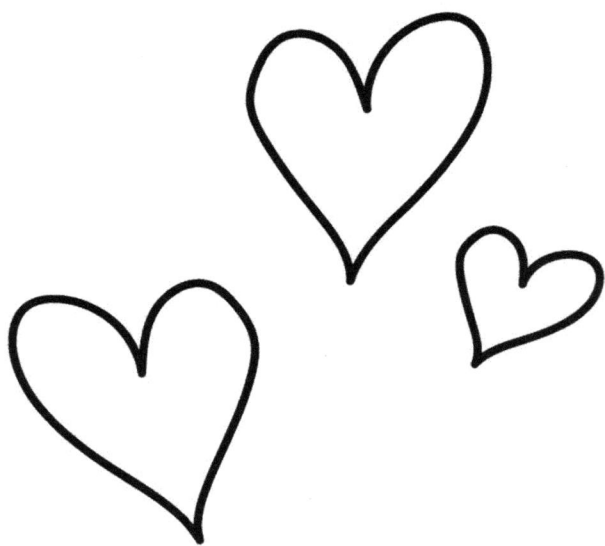

Hear

The next day, I woke up to the noisy alarm from my phone. I had set it for 6:00 a.m. so I could go for my next run because I had committed myself to just doing it and not thinking about it anymore. I wanted to show myself that I could do it, that I did love myself, and that I would continue to love myself every single day, not only on the days where I felt like exercising. I committed to every single day because I knew I was worthy, and I knew I wanted more joy and laughter in my life.

I noticed that after I moved my body, I could connect with it and my senses in a more intimate way. I could see and smell and taste and touch and hear everything around me, and I could use this information to understand myself and my life better. It felt as though life was talking to and through me using my senses.

This realization was followed by a phone call from a friend. I picked up the phone, and, while she talked to me about her experience the previous evening, I *heard* her very soft and joyful voice. I liked listening to her and to her voice. I was drawn to the softness in her. She noticed, too, and asked, "Can you hear how life is guiding us?" I smiled and said, "Yes. I'm noticing it, and I'm actually starting to enjoy it."

I hadn't known that this way of living was possible. Being so alive in every moment. I always used to think that this was too woo-woo for me, but it's not. It is simply being connected and present with yourself. If you think that this is not applicable to you, don't be afraid.

You are in the right place at the right time; everything comes in divine timing. When you open up your senses for yourself, you open up the senses for life, and that helps you to really feel and be with yourself in a more harmonious way. When you open up your senses and take in the beauty that you see and smell and taste and touch and hear all around you, then you are able to experience life in the way that it's supposed to be lived.

Touch

I can remember standing in front of the mirror and hating what I saw—myself and my body. I remember touching my stomach and being in such disharmony with myself that everything I said about myself and my body was negative. I had so many judgments and so much internalized shame that I made my body the problem, externalizing what I felt. When you hate your body, there's a difference between talking about loving your body and really loving and indulging in it. On my self-love journey, I realized that I could not possibly really love my body, touch it, and feel amazing in my skin if I was constantly criticizing it. How could I love myself from a place of hate? These two different behaviors can't fit together. I started to change this pattern by making a practice of standing in front of the mirror, looking at myself, and touching different parts of my body to consciously address that part of myself by noticing it and putting all my attention there. It felt like talking to a different human being.

This process became one of the most profound ways I could tune into my body and learn how to really and truly accept and love myself on a very deep level. I started to figure out where and what I was most afraid of, and I became honest about what I really didn't like about each body part. Instead of pushing all these body parts and thoughts away, I leaned into the feelings, accepting them so I could be present with them and with the magic that happened when I reconnected with all of my senses. Touch is one of the easiest and most gentle ways to show yourself and others love. I asked myself, "How do I want to be touched by me?" If I want to learn how to love myself, then I can't grab my tummy and talk negatively about it. I practiced conscious mirror work and exercises where I dimmed the light in a room and worshiped myself. Okay, at this point you may be laughing and wondering where this is going! But stick with me. I had similar thoughts about what I was doing because I didn't have anybody explaining self-love practices like this at the time. Nevertheless, the process felt very natural to me. It made me feel better about myself and look at my body more compassionately and with gratitude. This was a huge shift: I learned to slow down; to be present with myself; and to interact on a more conscious level with my body, addressing certain feelings that had been underneath all along.

I invite you to practice touching yourself with love and compassion. Practice what it feels like to be touched in the most loving, gentle, softest way possible; learn how to receive the feeling of touch. Acknowledge and honor yourself during this process. This is very important because when you learn what your body likes and what it doesn't like, how you want to be touched, in which way, what you like at what times, then you can set healthy boundaries and communicate to yourself and your partners and people around you what you need and what feels the most natural to you. You can also be touched by God, the divine, and life in a way that opens your heart.

When you are touched in a way that feels good to you, your body feels safe, which makes your nervous system feel safe. That, in turn, allows your body to be opened instead of shutting down. Establishing a sense of safety within your body is the most profound wisdom humans, especially women, can learn. Learn how to receive touch in a way that elevates you. When your body feels safe, the whole universe exhales. Having safety within your body is a state of being able to feel free and breathe in your soul; a state of expansion that allows you to let go of excess spiritual and emotional weight. From this place, you can let go of excess physical weight, too. *Please read that again.* When you establish a sense of safety within your body—through your nervous system, through touch that feels good to you—you allow your body to stop holding onto what has been keeping you hidden, such as excess weight, and your body can finally feel safe enough to stop hiding. This will allow it to shape itself in a gentle way. This is sustainable weight loss because it comes from love, not fear.

This is one of the keys on your journey toward self-love and the connection to losing weight once and for all. I want you to congratulate yourself for being open and for making it this far because this is how you receive all the blessings and abundance that are yours in this life. You're now open to the most amazing love story of your life.

So how can you learn to give and receive touch in a way that's filled with pleasure, joy, and fun? I want you to go into your kitchen. I want you to find a fruit or a vegetable. Maybe it is an orange, an apple, a banana, or a pepper—something yummy. I want you to feel it in your hand. Now, combine all your senses—the seeing, the smelling, the tasting, the hearing, and the touching. Touch the fruit or vegetable in a way you've never touched it before. I want you to imagine it being a partner, someone you really, really love. You may even have romantic feelings for it! Yes, I can see you smiling and laughing. You're not crazy. Enjoy the process of having fun with your fruit or vegetable. Look at it through the lens of love. How would somebody touch this amazing fruit or vegetable with all their senses? I want you to close your eyes and touch the skin on the outside. How does it feel? How does your hand feel? Notice the point where the skin of the food touches your skin. Notice the connection. Bring it toward your mouth. Try to touch it with your lips in a way that feels good to you. How does your skin feel? What is happening inside your body? You can combine all your senses. What do you hear, smell, see, touch, and taste? This is a process of learning how to really indulge yourself, becoming one with the Creator and with all creations. Eating is an intimate process of feeding yourself, an act of devotion to yourself and your wellness. Eating nourishes not only your body but also your soul. Eating is sexy!

CHAPTER 3

ENERGY

Nutrition and Hydration

You know that hydration is good for you, but how do you make yourself drink enough water during the day, every day? One thing that helped me was having a big water bottle that I carried around with me everywhere. Buy yourself a beautiful water bottle to take with you (or put an inspiring sticker on one you already have). You can spice up the water itself, too. If you spice up food to make it more pleasing, why shouldn't you do it with your water?! It doesn't have to be boring to be healthy. Water can taste good. Put a slice of orange, lemon, or lime into your water. Use mint, cucumbers, or berries in it. Make your water sexy. It is easier to do things that are good for you when you actually like them!

I know it sounds a little bit silly, but set an alarm clock to help you drink more water. Setting alarms throughout the day can help you to reconnect with your body's needs. A quick reminder to focus on drinking enough water also helps temper cravings, which is a very important part of weight loss. In general, if you feel hungry all the time or if you crave certain food, like sugar, there's often a need underneath that is not fulfilled. So every single time you crave something, ask yourself, "Why do I want to eat right now? Is it because I'm physically hungry or am I emotionally hungry? Is there something that I need to address? Is there some emotional need that demands my attention right now?" When you tune into yourself and your body, you become more aware. You can meet your own needs and expect less from the world outside, which will allow you to feel a sense of control over life. In this way, you can be a better human being for other people, and you can show up with more energy for your family, for your children, for your partner. You can show up at work in a different way. You can fulfill your purpose in a deeper way.

Taking care of yourself means being connected to yourself and having more energy to experience life with all of your senses awakened. Being self-focused isn't bad, and it doesn't make you selfish. It's important that you rewire your brain and learn what it means to truly love yourself and honor your needs and not feel guilty about it. There is nothing wrong with feeling good; life is meant to feel good. And your body is the vehicle through which you experience life. The more you see your body as a vessel for experience, the more you will allow your soul and light to shine from the inside.

Next up is the "welcome home" portion of your journey. You want to welcome in all the beautiful, nutritious foods and flavors that are here on Earth for you to eat to radiate your light. These foods and flavors have been given to you to find pleasure.

Managing food is a very big part of your everyday life. Maybe you're someone who's done detox program after detox program and tried all the diets and latest weightloss trends. I, too, tried every diet under the sun, every tool and trick in the book; I even traveled around the globe to learn from trainers how to lose weight. Everything worked for a short while. But the process of focusing too much attention—obsessing, really—on my weight and restrictions pushed me in a different direction. Maybe I lost weight on the outside for a couple of months or even years, but it always came back. No matter how much or how little food I ate, nothing changed on the inside. The key to self-love and loving the body you're in isn't changing the way your body looks; it's changing the way you see food. It's a radical change to see food in a new and more joyful way.

Changing the way you see food is forgetting about calories, points, and colors—it's forgetting about what food does to the body and, instead, focusing on what food does for the soul. Teach yourself to find joy in food; indulge in every bite; and express gratitude for the pleasure of food. This is how you create radical transformation, *true* transformation, inside and out. For free resources about effective methods to change your relationship with food, visit **carolineeickhoff.com/free**.

For most of my life, people told me that I would never lose the weight I wanted to lose because everyone in my family is big, overweight, and struggles with diabetes, insulin, or cancer. Even my doctors told me that I couldn't lose weight because I have big bones and a slow metabolism. I also was diagnosed with a metabolic syndrome, a combination of different things that made it impossible for me to lose weight. Maybe you have had a similar experience, fighting off the thoughts and opinions of other people, fighting against attaching those labels to your body. Right now, I really want you to tune those voices out and tune in to yourself, into your body and your heart, and listen to your own inner voice. That's what I did for myself, and now I can say that, even after being diagnosed with type 2 diabetes, after listening to all those expert opinions, I still lost the weight. And here I am, 130 pounds lighter in the end. Those labels didn't stick because I wouldn't let them.

I needed to take my power back, power over my body and food, and give myself and my inner knowing more credit than the outside opinions. I made an effort to keep learning so that I could become the happy woman I wanted to be. Even before I lost the weight, I made a decision to eat without guilt and to eat in a way that made me feel joyful. It felt as though I was making a deal with my soul and God because He told me, "If you only listen to my voice and you keep going based on what I'm going to tell you, you will receive everything you have been yearning for. You will be the size you long to be and look the way you want to look. I need you to be in a body that supports your bigger vision. I need you to be in a body that is nurtured and healthy because you have big things to do. I need you to shine my light on this road." Yes, God really taught me these things, and, despite not knowing where to start, I trusted Him and took small steps over and over again until I was able to see food as love, to make food that felt like love, and to let go of the torment I had experienced in my relationship with food for so long.

Microbiome

A microbiome is a collection of all the microbes, such as bacteria, viruses, and their genes, that naturally live in and on your body. There are certain bacteria you can't live without, and it's very important to have a healthy microbiome for health and overall wellness. Happy starts on the inside with a happy microbiome! There are simple ways to strengthen your microbiome: avoid processed foods as much as possible and increase your intake of probiotics and prebiotics, such as those in gut-friendly fermented foods like milk, kefir, and miso. Fennel, asparagus, potatoes, onions, garlic, leeks, broth, and prebiotic vegetables are amazing ways you can support your body's natural immunity.

Sleep

Taking care of yourself and your energy must be accompanied by taking care of your sleep. Unless you provide your body with adequate time for restoration and rejuvenation, all the other work you do to look after yourself will be for naught. Sleep is the time your body utilizes the nutrition you have provided to repair tissues and improve muscle growth. Allowing your body to do this work is crucial to your health and well-being journey.

THE SECRET OF FOOD

It is important to note that not all sleep is created equally. There are different types of sleep, and each stage serves a different purpose. A healthy sleep cycle includes non-rapid eye movement (or NREM) sleep and rapid eye movement (or REM) sleep. NREM sleep is responsible for light sleep, physical restoration, and growth hormone release. REM sleep, associated with vivid dreams, is responsible for cognitive restoration. This is the sleep that helps you feel mentally rejuvenated. Poor sleep quality is responsible for not only physical exhaustion, but mental exhaustion, too.

How do you set yourself up for healthy sleep?

First, align your food intake with your sleep needs. I often used to eat food very late at night. Then I struggled to sleep afterward because my body was so focused on digestion. At other times, I stopped eating at 4:00 p.m. and went to bed with hunger cravings and stomach pain because I was so undernourished. Food impacts your sleep, and sleep impacts every aspect of your life. So learning to properly eat to protect your sleep is vital for loving your body and loving your life.

But even if you consume food at ideal times, you may still wake up in the morning and feel exhausted, wanting to crawl back into bed again. How can you wake up and feel revitalized and energized, ready for the day, and able to take care of your body's needs throughout that day? It starts the night before. I set an alarm on my alarm clock (not my phone!) one hour before bedtime to remind me it's time to put my phone away. I do not check any social media or do any scrolling of any kind after that alarm goes off!

Moreover, putting away the screens halts my absorption of blue light. The blue light from screens affects melatonin, a hormone naturally produced from the amino acid tryptophan by your pineal gland in response to darkness.

The pineal gland produces this hormone to regulate your sleep-wake cycle over a twenty-four-hour period. Melatonin levels increase in the evening when it gets dark outside, which promotes drowsiness and signals the body to prepare for sleep. The blue light from screens, however, inhibits the production of melatonin, disrupting this natural sleep-wake cycle. Here are some tips to naturally boost melatonin.

- Get sunlight.
- Eat tryptophan-rich foods, such as meat products and dairy.
- Take a warm bath.
- Limit artificial light (put screens away before you go to bed).

When my wake-up alarm rings in the morning, I choose to start my day with stillness, being present in the day and with myself, rather than looking at my phone or laptop as soon as I wake up. Carefully considering how you spend your evening and early morning screen time will promote healthier sleep patterns and overall well-being.

The processes of winding down and coming back to center, going to bed with diligence and waking up with diligence, will calm your mind and body. They ensure you get good quality sleep at night. And good quality sleep will enhance your immune function, digestion, bone formation, production of new cells, and blood pressure.

Proper sleep also keeps your endocrine system functioning optimally. In addition to melatonin, this system produces seven other primary hormones: insulin, estrogen, progesterone, prolactin, testosterone, serotonin, and cortisol. These hormones travel through your bloodstream from one part of the body to another, helping to control how cells and organs do their work, including your metabolism. There are foods you can eat that help support your endocrine system, especially if you want to feel vibrant, young, and beautiful! Understanding these seven main hormones your body produces, as well as their functions, is a great way to work toward your self-love goals.

When I was overweight, I felt as though I was constantly fighting against my body and that it was always under attack. Turns out, when insulin and cortisol levels are chronically high, it's very hard to lose weight. Cortisol and insulin play a significant role in metabolism and fat storage. Chronically high cortisol levels lead to increased appetite, cravings, and the accumulation of abdominal fat. High cortisol levels also disrupt other hormones involved in weight regulation, such as insulin, which further contributes to difficulty losing weight. It becomes impossible to lose weight, even if you eat salad the whole day. I am sure you are aware of the phenomenon of not eating and still not losing weight; in fact, you likely gain weight. This is because the body is too stressed to let go. It is under constant pressure to fight and survive. When you are able to regulate your hormone levels, your body is more likely to be healthy and fit.

I made huge progress in losing weight, keeping it off, and falling in love with myself when I supported my body in the best way I possibly could. Having knowledge about the purpose of hormones helped me to stop fighting against my body and, instead, understand what it needed to move in the same direction as ease, joy, and health. I felt as though I had the power to reprogram my system to work for me and not against me.

When I lost the weight, my diabetes and insulin resistance reversed themselves and my receptor cells could function properly again. Consequently, I didn't have hunger cravings all the time; my sleep was better; my digestion and gut health normalized; my sex drive came back; and I was happy. Finally, my body felt like a place I wanted to be!

Move Your Body

Learning to move my body in the right way took some time. I used to be so ashamed of my body that I couldn't even go to the gym. I was so afraid of doing the wrong thing, of being embarrassed and looking like a fool, that I didn't even bother trying. So I started small, walking outside, and, to be honest, that was amazing for me. I really enjoyed my morning walks because they helped me to do something for my body that naturally felt good, and I didn't put pressure on myself to feel a certain way or look a certain way—I just went with how I felt while doing it. It also didn't make my joints hurt, so I enjoyed the process of finding the right movement for my body.

Maybe you are in this situation right now, where you want to start moving your body in a way that feels good again, in a way that's good for you. Maybe your body has become an object of shame for you, and you don't know how to move it with love. I want to remind you that your body is a temple; it is the vessel from which all life is experienced—all beauty, joy, and pleasure. You are allowed to move your body in whatever way feels good to you. You are allowed to take up space in the room, on the sidewalk, in the ocean, in the world. Find the space where your body wants to move, where your body feels the most peace, where you feel fluid. Be careful not to overdo it in the beginning because every single time you do something new and move your body in a way that you haven't before, your body listens and reacts, so speak gently.

When I first started coming back from my short walks, my body was sore because I was moving it in a way I hadn't before. I had to take it slowly, one step at a time, honoring my body and listening to what it could manage each time. Staying tuned in to my body was a very important part of the movement journey because even movement can be used to numb and escape emotions. I needed to make sure that I wasn't using movement as the next binge, as the next distraction, so I had to become present with every part of my body while I moved, listening to what felt good and what made me feel strong.

Start with movement for your body, not against your body. Every decision you make about food, about new routines or action steps, should lead to making you feel good and valued. Overstepping your boundaries and going to extremes is always a push against yourself, not for yourself. If you keep pushing your body beyond what is kind and what it can manage on a given day, you will burn out in the long run and lose any progress you have made. You need to be stable and integrate a consistent routine into your life that fits your lifestyle, that fits your body, and that you really enjoy doing because you will only continue doing the things you really enjoy in the long run. When life happens, and it will, when you feel stressed and everything seems out of control, you will prioritize what feels good to you when it's time to take care of yourself. Movement that feels stressful will only amplify your stress, so don't set yourself up for failure. Be prepared to not lose motivation during stressful times; don't chase the perfect workout or the strictest exercise regime. It's unrealistic to repeat those when you are under pressure. Movement is about going with the flow, coming back to the rituals that you are learning about in this book to stay on track and to use consistent, aligned action for yourself, from a place of love.

Increasing your flexibility is another valuable way to love your body and mind. Stretching allows you to feel the different muscle groups in your body; it invites you to slow down and connect with every part of you that carries you through this world. It requires mental flexibility, encouraging you to be present with your body and challenge yourself to feel and experience manageable discomfort and not give up. Stretching also helps your muscles to recover after exercise and stimulates energy circulation throughout your body.

Stretching can be sitting down on your mat, extending your legs, and trying to touch your toes; first your left and then your right toes. I invite you to do this practice from a place of love;

be gentle with yourself and allow your body time to stretch and adjust to this new growth. The key is not to move and stretch because you hate yourself or you hate your body, but because you find joy in the movements that make you fit. Slow and steady wins the race.

I would like you to put on the song that you picked for yourself in Chapter 1, and I want you to start playing the song loudly and moving your body at the same time. Maybe, if it helps you to feel more comfortable, close your eyes and allow your body to feel the music. It's all about the feeling. You will realize very quickly that the body moves itself, so allow yourself to express your truth through it. Feeling the music through your body can become a ritual for you to step into energy during your everyday life; to go from being to doing. Energy is flow, stepping out of chaos and into calm. You need to move stagnant energy through your body in order to be present and alive. Use this time for yourself and honor your body by moving it, not from your mind, but from a centered heart space. Suspend your thoughts about the movement and just move.

Self-Care NOW

I know all too well how busy life can get and how many intrusions can demand your attention on any given day. Self-care is an aspect of well-being that needs to be prioritized and practiced in order to reap its benefits and achieve a happy and fulfilled life. Yes, life can become very stressful, but taking time to reflect on your needs, even if it's only for a moment, is very important. What do you need right now? Do you need

ENERGY

something to drink? Do you need something to eat? Do you need to take a deep breath? It is these simple moments that make a huge difference over time because you need to become a person who cares for yourself. You can't do everything for everybody else and then burn out and have nothing left for you in the end. It is these simple self-loving moments and pockets of time that you must create for yourself to be with yourself in the here and now. Making time for yourself and taking care of yourself in those small moments is essential to ensure you don't need to take more time later on just to get your energy back.

It takes more time to get sick and then get back on track than it does to keep yourself healthy. When you live with a self-care mindset, your thoughts, your beliefs, and your actions determine your well-being.
- How can you love yourself in a way that supports your bigger vision?
- How can you love yourself even through intense emotions and not shy away from them?
- How can you be with yourself in the midst of chaos?

These are the answers that determine how your life unfolds.

I know what it's like to feel as though you just don't have the time. I've been there. You, too, are trying to do your best, trying to take care of everybody and be there for everybody else, making them a priority and forgetting about yourself. This self-love journey is about being there for yourself and doing the best you can do for others without losing yourself at the same time. It is possible to do it all and have it all. Maybe it doesn't look the way you think it's supposed to look, but that doesn't mean it's wrong. And it can be even simpler than you think.

Self-care is not a fleeting trend; it is a commitment to nurturing your own mental, emotional, and physical well-being. It is a deliberate act of self-love, a reminder that you and your needs are important. Whether it's setting aside time for yourself, nourishing your body with wholesome food, or taking time out in nature, self-care practices will allow you to hear the voice of your innermost self and to understand who you are and what your purpose is in this world. The practice of self-care is more than just the act of spending time with yourself; it is about discovering how you feel and who you are when all the noise and distractions are stripped away.

Now, take out your phone and open up your calendar. I want you to schedule a date with yourself and your own thoughts. It can be a tiny window of only 30 minutes or a whole day. It's up to you. Trying to do something when you don't have the time to do it never works out, especially if it's for yourself. So be practical. Find ways to make time for yourself so that you can be present with what is going on inside your body and in your life to discover what you need. It can be very uncomfortable in the beginning, and it can feel very unnatural to just sit and do nothing and be with yourself, but this is exactly the point. Stop running from task to task; slow your life down so you can actually listen to yourself, so that your soul can finally breathe and feel free to express itself. The state you exist in with yourself is as important as an appointment you have with other people because you are the first person you meet everyday. You have to make yourself a priority over and over again and remind yourself of how amazing you are and that what you are doing in this world is amazing. Filling up your own cup is not selfish. It's the most beautiful thing you can do for yourself and the people around you. Visit **carolineickhoff.com/free** to learn more about filling your own cup.

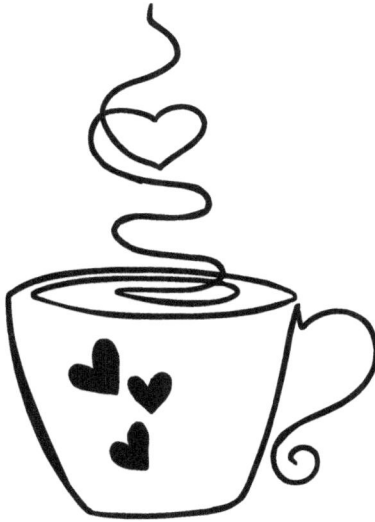

CHAPTER 4

CREATION

Create Your Reality Through Your Thoughts

Now that you understand the secret to creating a life of love and making your dream life a reality, turn your thoughts to what I call the *reality loop*.

So what is the *reality loop*? It is a loop where your thoughts create your emotions and your emotions create your thoughts. Thoughts lead to certain behaviors. Repeating the behavior is a pattern; the patterns become habits; and the habits become your personality. The result of these patterns either makes you happy or creates other emotions that lead to particular thoughts, and these thoughts then lead to behaviors, then habits, then emotions again. This is the loop. It can spiral upward or downward depending on the thoughts. How and what do you think about yourself, about your life, and about your food on a regular basis?

To create an internal environment where you can thrive, you need to build momentum with your thoughts.

I first started shifting my life when I realized how important it is to actively stop negative mental spiraling by changing and shifting my thoughts. Magic happens when you become aware of the power you have to create your own life on your own terms. And it all starts with what you believe about yourself, what you choose to believe about the world, and what you choose to believe about your life—right here and right now. Your actual thoughts can lead to new experiences that open your life and allow you to partake in the abundance of all that surrounds you. Or your thoughts can work against you and create limits on what you can achieve.

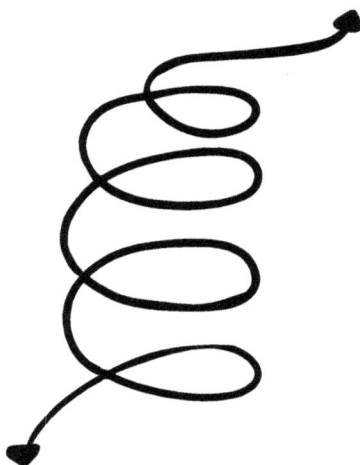

Now that you have the awareness that thoughts have the power to create emotional changes and a peaceful internal state, you can choose thoughts that align with your bigger vision. How? First, let go of thoughts that belittle you ... that keep you small. You likely adopted these thoughts in childhood from the environment that you grew up in. They are thoughts and patterns that your parents modeled. As an adult, you will continue to choose these thoughts until you reach a point where you want and are ready for a different outcome. Then, you will actively choose new thoughts about your life and how you think about yourself, your body, your food, and your health. You can *choose* what you want to think about yourself and what feels good and supports you.

The thoughts you choose will determine tomorrow's results. If you think that you are not worthy of X, Y, or Z, you will not be it or have it. If you think that you are worthy, your entire being will start looking for ways to bring what you want into your reality. When you think that you will never be able to lose the weight, that will be your reality. The universe will respond: "And so it is." When you open yourself up and make yourself available to a new reality, you flip the game.

Human beings must live according to their nature, and when you live in accordance with this nature, you live in flow—allowing life to unfold organically. I believe the nature of humans is to live in joy, bliss, happiness, health, abundance, and light. This is who humans truly are. So changing your thoughts is actually a process of remembering—remembering who you are and what you have been created for; remembering what your true nature is, coming back to your truth. When you remember what is underneath the thoughts that keep you in destructive patterns, you will be guided to choose thoughts that align with your truth. Thoughts that keep you distracted and focused on what is outside of you keep you away from your destiny and a life of love.

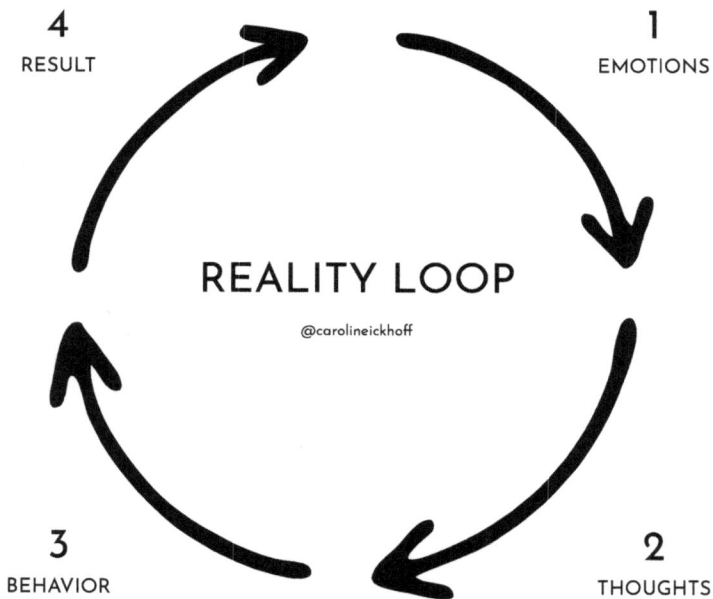

4 RESULT

1 EMOTIONS

REALITY LOOP

@carolineickhoff

3 BEHAVIOR

2 THOUGHTS

Who currently controls your thoughts? Strange question, right? Consider that you are not only your conscious mind, but also a combination of many versions of yourself as a child, all of whom have different needs. And yes, I mean that you have more than one inner child! These versions of you have developed based on your lived experiences, your trauma, your upbringing, and your beliefs. This is why the work and the self-love journey isn't straight; it's a journey that will take loops and turns and lead you where you never expected to go.

You have different needs at different times based on the situations you are in. This is true for your thoughts as well. Your thoughts are a reflection of what is going on inside. When you think, "I want to be healthy," and you aren't, it could be because there is a part of you that is afraid of being skinny because it feels too vulnerable. It doesn't feel safe to be in a smaller body. Maybe you find safety in your bigger body because you believe you won't have to get too close to people. And, perhaps, this keeps you safe from being hurt. I invite you to open up to this concept because your unfulfilled desires are usually blocked by a part of you that is resistant to that very desire. If this weren't true, that desire would be met. But it's not. So ask yourself, "Why not?"

While this exercise can be frustrating, it can also be a relief to find out that some part of you is sabotaging the whole because that means you have the power to stop the sabotage and finally achieve your dreams. The work that I did to free myself from the fear of losing weight was what helped me to finally lose the weight. I stopped hiding and stepped into my power and owned it. When I was on my journey, at first I thought that my goal was to have a different body—as though that would solve everything. But the more I explored myself, the more I meditated, the more time I spent in nature, the more silent I became, and the more I observed my thoughts, the more I discovered parts of me that were afraid of being seen. Maybe you feel this way, too.

Revealing these hidden parts of yourself can feel very confrontational. It's difficult to honestly admit that part of you wants to undermine your own goals. So it's important that you do this kind of introspection in a gentle and loving way. If you truly want to live in a body with a purpose, feel peace about who you are, and live a life that actually matters to you, you must get clear about the intentions behind your decisions. To understand your decisions, you need to understand your thoughts and the power they have over your emotions and behaviors. This is the game changer.

When I discovered the parts of me that wanted to hide, I realized that these parts were afraid to own my power. They rebelled against the parts of me that wanted to lose weight because these parts believed that there was a benefit to being a human in a bigger body. There was a little girl inside me that didn't feel safe anywhere but in the body I was in.

As you start to discover these different aspects of yourself, it's important to listen to what they have to say and to give them what they need to feel safe. When you start to feel safe in every part of you, you will be able to integrate them into a healthy whole and move your life and your body in the direction of love and health.

Play this little game to cultivate the love you want to feel for yourself. Ask yourself these questions:
- How do I benefit from not having my dreams come true right now?
- How do I benefit from not losing weight, from not becoming successful, from not being in love?

- What do I fear will happen if I achieve this goal right now?
- What would I need to give up in order to achieve it?

Notice how you answer these questions. Listen to what your mind is telling you. When you can answer these questions honestly, you will open yourself up to thoughts that bring about the happy, fulfilled life you seek—a life where your wildest dreams come true and you discover your purpose. For additional free materials on cultivating self-love through thought, visit **carolineickhoff.com/free**. Change your thoughts and you will change your world. I promise.

Beliefs

One of the best messages I ever received from God was: "You can never outwork your identity." Beliefs and what you believe to be true are the most important aspects of your character:
- With what or whom do you identify?
- What do you believe about yourself on a regular basis?
- What do you want to believe about your body?

These are the important questions that you need to ask yourself when creating your reality through your thoughts. At first, you may only identify with basic characteristics: "My name is Carolin. This is my profession. I live in this town. I like mangoes and the ocean. I love to be at the beach. I like cooking and my favorite food is lasagna." But magic happens when you go even deeper and get to the core of who you are with the really important questions:

- Who am I truly?
- Who is it that is asking these questions?
- Why am I here?
- What is my purpose?

The more I asked myself these questions, the more I loved myself and walked in my purpose. The more I loved myself and walked in my purpose, the more energized I felt. From this state, life force could flow through me.

The process of becoming better is about actively stripping away all the layers and masks that you think define you by questioning yourself. Again and again, you will peel back layers until you reach the divine—whether you call it nature, life, God, or the source, whatever feels true for you—where you start to understand that there is something bigger, a higher power that makes the grass grow, that creates the seasons, that has the power to make your heart beat even when you're not thinking about it. This is the most loving awareness that there is in the universe, and you are a part of it.

Express gratitude for yourself and for how far you have come on this journey because you have discovered the peace that is available to you simply for being you. There is a loving source that wants you to know you are worthy just for being here. Many people can't accept this because society is programmed to believe that they have to work very hard for everything. But I don't believe this is our natural state as human beings. You will burn out from putting on all these masks because you can't keep up with the masquerade. These masks will make you sick because you are not doing and being who you truly are.

Remove these masks, one by one, like the petals of a rose that open slowly to reveal splendor. This is what I call rose medicine—like the thoughts, behaviors, and characteristics that no longer serve you, let one petal fall at a time. Allow peace to fill their place. This is how you come back to your core, to the center of who you are, to the loving awareness, the splendor of the rose that is you. For me, it is a golden ball inside this beautiful flower. That's why I created the Love Ball, to give you permission to give yourself the attention you deserve and to remember that you are divine.

LOVE BALL

Actions

Now that you are starting to know who you truly are, it is your job and your responsibility to act. The next step is a profound process of taking action from a place of love instead of taking action from a place of unworthiness. It is a process of taking action from a place of already being good enough, already being beautiful, already being amazing. That is the frequency and energetic space you want to take action from. This is the exact point that determines whether you make it through to the next season or you fall back into old patterns. I call it the ripple effect of love. If you start with love, what radiates out will be rooted in love, and this will allow you to take actions that align with love. If the action starts from a place of punishment, the ripple effects will be rooted in fear and hate and will not align with who you truly are.

The minute you take action from a place of love, you will enter a place that is golden. A place that is bright and light and beautiful. You don't have to prove yourself to anyone anymore. You don't have to yearn or do anything to be worthy of love. When you flip the script and seek out what you are already worthy of, you can support your body to enjoy the pleasures of being alive.

Compare this to taking action from a place of restriction. You can repeat a habit every day, or you can take action from a place of abundance. You can live with a scarcity mindset—not enough love, not enough food, not enough money—or you can take action from a mindset of abundance: "There is more than enough, and I am allowed to have some." This mindset will determine your outcome.

Writing this book was an action—one that I wrote from a mindset of abundance. I wrote part of this book in Laguna Beach, California. Something came alive in that amazing setting, and everything came from a place of love, supercharged with the intention of purity.

As I sat in the sun, my cheeks glowing because I was filled with Mother Nature and all her beauty, I felt so blessed and vibrant because my whole body relaxed, and my channel opened to receive the purest form of love for you, my reader. There were majestic mountains, green and large, lining the horizon. Next to them was the ocean, an oasis of pure joy. It was so calming. I couldn't tell where the ocean ended with the water touching the sky. The birds chirped in the background; nature spoke. And I cried because I realized that I had flipped the script on my life. Everything flowed from a place of love, a place of abundance.

I had decided to live a life worth living; I had committed and dedicated myself to serve humanity in its purest form. Reflecting right in that moment made me smile because I would never have imagined myself sitting there talking about my story that had caused me so much pain—pain that I had turned into a message. You can do the same. You can transcend any negative emotion or situation that you may be experiencing. If I can transform all of my pain and self-loathing, it's possible for you, too. I am so happy that you have decided to experience life in all its abundance. Acting from a place of love leads to a place of love, but it's not a place. It is a legacy.

Start taking action today. Cultivate an abundance mindset by developing a gratitude practice. By consciously acknowledging and appreciating the abundance already present in your life—whether it's the love of family and friends, the beauty of nature, or the simple pleasures of everyday food—you will open your heart to receive even more blessings.

Another way to embody love in your daily life is through compassionate communication. By speaking and listening from a place of empathy, understanding, and respect, you foster deeper connections with those around you, cultivating an atmosphere of trust, authenticity, and mutual support. Whether it's offering words of encouragement to a friend in need, expressing appreciation to a loved one, or simply being present and attentive in your interactions, your words and actions have the power to uplift, inspire, and transform lives.

Celebration

Let's celebrate the realization of how far you've come, of how far you have stretched yourself. Let's celebrate every little thing in your life because most people wait for a life-changing event before they start to celebrate who they are or what they have accomplished. Waiting until you have lost all the weight and only then celebrating yourself is the wrong way around. You must celebrate yourself for everything you already are, for everything you are discovering about yourself right now. Celebrate being brave enough to go on this journey and being brave enough to venture into unexplored parts of yourself. And celebrate the little wins. It all starts with these small steps that you take every day to honor yourself from a place of love and show yourself that you care.

You can honor yourself by finding "I am" phrases that feel good to you and that you can truly believe—this is key. If you are saying, "I am super skinny, and I love it," but you don't believe it, there is a discrepancy in your energetic field. You want to avoid this. Instead, speak things that all your parts inside and outside believe and that you can truly say out loud. When I first started on my self-love journey, I focused on one part of my body that I could genuinely say I loved. I said, "I am brave for walking this journey. What do I like about myself? I like how my pinky finger looks because it always reminds me of the pinky promise I made to myself and my soul that I would finish what I started."

Now, when I look at my pinky finger, I remember my promise to myself; it's a powerful reminder of self-love. Keeping the promises you make to yourself and celebrating all the little wins that you achieve on a regular basis are radical acts of self-love. They can take the form of celebrating yourself for drinking enough water, for buying yourself flowers, for journaling three times in a row, for going for a walk every single day in a given week. When you keep celebrating the small wins, when they become your new normal, they become a habit, and you forget how difficult they once were. So always remember where you came from, remember what you have already achieved, and remember to praise yourself for even the most ordinary win. This is how you celebrate yourself from a place of love and from a place of purity.

CHAPTER 5
RELATIONSHIPS

Be Your Own Best Friend

You can celebrate yourself right now by putting on your favorite song and dancing to it because you are becoming the creator of your own dream life! You know how to take actions that are in alignment with your higher purpose, and, now, it's time to focus on your foundations—empathy, gentle compassion for yourself, forgiveness, and kindness. These are virtues that you have to learn, practice, and master in order to experience heaven on Earth.

Before you can find honest connections with other people and enter relationships that help you thrive, you must first establish a kind and honest relationship with yourself. And to be kind and honest with yourself, you need to practice patience. The patience to know that your present life doesn't determine your future, that God is ultimately in control, and that He will decide when the right doors need to be opened. Exercise patience with your body as it heals from all the years of self-loathing and self-abuse; do not expect it to fix itself in two or three months. Be patient with yourself, and become your own best friend first. This includes befriending your body just as it is in this moment. Be compassionate to yourself and know that you are trying your best.

Everything that is coming into your life is good for you, moving you in the direction of God's purpose for your life. These practices of patience and empathy will lead to ultimate freedom. It is never too late to start. It's never too late to get back on track. It is always the perfect timing because the timing is always now. God knows exactly where He wants you to be; it is your job to be receptive to His nudges and His voice. Being your own best friend also means practicing all the steps that you have learned in this book: the real talk, engaging your senses, raising your energy, and becoming the creation so that you can shine from the inside out.

The relationship with yourself must flow from knowing who you truly are and being comfortable with yourself in this space. Owning the essence of you is now a pivotal point in your journey because you are going to fall, and the only way to hold space for your fallible self is to be comfortable with who you are. You are so used to avoiding falling that you must learn to repeatedly fall with grace because you are only human. Imagine you are with your best friend who shares with you that they have done something that they feel deep shame about. What would you say to them? How would you encourage them? What would you do? You wouldn't shame your best friend; you wouldn't break them down. This is how you must approach yourself, how you must love yourself, too. Becoming a living embodiment of what you stand for means practicing showing up for yourself over and over again in grace. It's not easy to empathize and be kind to yourself, but you must make it a habit to build a relationship with yourself first.

Take a moment right now to review the previous chapters and any notes you took or any journal entries you wrote while reading. Did you make any commitments to yourself that you're not yet doing?

- What can you kick-start today without blaming yourself for not starting sooner?
- What can you do right now to be your own best friend?
- Does your body need a nap or a walk?
- Do you need to eat the whole chocolate bar, or do you need to drink two glasses of water and cook yourself a nutritious meal made with an abundance of superfoods?
- What does it look like to be your own best friend?
- What triggers a "yes?"
- What guilts you into a "yes" when you truly mean "no?"
- What is it that you truly want from this process of prioritizing yourself?

For me, it was writing this book. I told myself that I didn't have time to write; my mind focused on all the other things that I needed to do instead. It convinced me that my story was not important and that people probably wouldn't even read it, but my soul was craving the truth. And I know that I always have to follow these nudges because whenever I go through the fear to the other side, there is always true freedom in the end. I've learned that magic happens when you go right into the storm rather than run from it. Don't pretend to not notice that there is a storm and distract yourself from your own truth, from the longing inside to be heard and seen. There is a place inside you that is craving the truth of who you really are.

I am supported by life because I'm sitting in my own vision board. I'm not exaggerating when I say you can create your own reality. What will happen if everything you want really comes true? If you really lose all the weight, if you really become successful, what will happen? You will realize abundance. But I find that you have to practice your success and prepare your body and your nervous system to hold all the abundance, all the love and joy there is to hold. You must prepare your body to let the love flow through you.

It is important that you learn how to be proud of yourself and make it a regular habit to notice everything you have achieved. You have been created to soar. Ask yourself, "When was the first time I decided not to fly?" There was a time in my life where I felt like a chicken sitting in a cage. And when you grow up like that, like a chicken sitting in a cage talking about being able to fly, it becomes normal to stay in the cage, to do what you've been told to do, to keep yourself trapped. Now, with all the knowledge and awareness that you are gaining, remember that you're not a chicken. You are a bird who can fly. The cage is open, not closed. You can step outside of your self-created cage. It has been open the whole time. Step out of that cage and fly.

You have the power to make the decision to not stay in the cage any longer. You have the power to let go of what you are holding so tightly, to open your hands and release, to let go of what is weighing you down, and fly. Give yourself permission to be the embodiment of your own freedom because, if you stay in places where you don't belong, you will never truly be happy. Stand up, rise up, spread your wings, and be the person you have always wanted to be. By deciding who you are, you become that person. You cannot put a price on this kind of relationship.

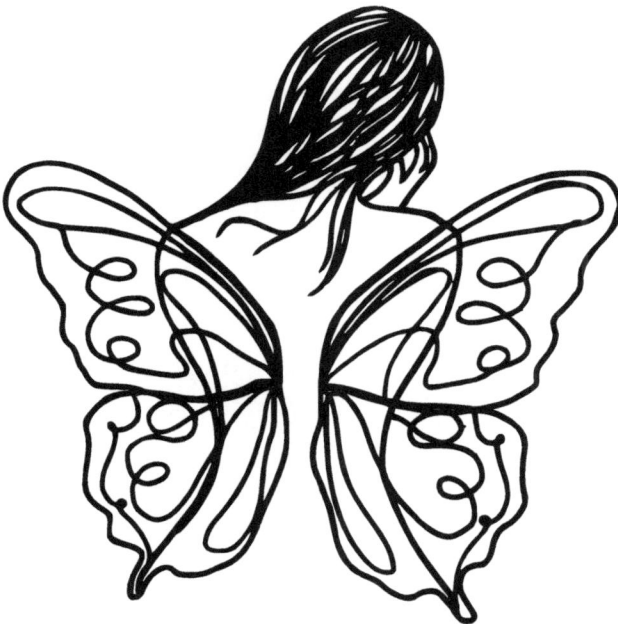

Family

You hold much wisdom inside you already, and you always have access to your higher source to gain even more to understand yourself and your life. Part of this wisdom includes understanding your family and where you have come from. Now that you are able to show yourself compassion and access your higher source, you can practice grace for any difficult family relationships. Practicing patience and forgiveness with your family may be your greatest challenge yet as family may cause the most pain. But you are here to become the master of your own life, the lover of your own life, and your family relationships can illuminate what you still need to work on and face in yourself. Likewise, you can be an example to them of what is possible, what healing power and joy awaits if one is willing to be brave.

It is amazing to see what happens when you are willing to release the judgment and shame that you have been holding on to for so many years when you practice the purity of your intentions. I invite you to focus on where you place your attention. Do you talk negatively about your family? Can you practice being more patient, kind, and compassionate? Often, negative patterns are intergenerational; your parents learned certain patterns modeled by their parents and then repeated them in your childhood, such as keeping secrets, substance abuse, and not talking about emotions. Nobody could teach the next generation how to do things differently, so it became a cycle. Your parents were children once, and it is likely that their emotions and dreams were shoved down and pushed aside by their own parents. Everyone is doing the best they can with what they have and where they're coming from.

It's interesting to try to see your parents from this perspective because some of the pain you're carrying around may be because they didn't know how to do better, and their parents didn't know how to do better, and so on. The cycle continues until somebody is ready to stand up and say, "Enough. No more." The cycle ends when somebody is ready to change, to do something different, something that has never been done in that family before. This is an open circle; there is a way out. You have been given this family, these patterns, to grow out of, to heal, to transcend the pain and show others the way out. And the way out of this generational cycle is not by blaming or shaming but by practicing being your own best friend—by giving yourself what your family was never able to give you—so that you can find peace and show them compassion instead of blame.

Now, you can choose to shift your perspective.
• What do you want to see?
• What do you want to do with this knowledge?
• What if you can do this for yourself?

Life is not against you; it is always for you. It is a loving awareness that wants you to be a greater force for good in this world, but you can only be the greatest force for good if you know and are willing to experience contrast. Give yourself and your family members time to reflect on who you *and* they are. This is an internal process, a time to reflect and digest. A time to practice patience.

This is an example of the desires God puts into the hearts of people so they can bring them to life. The more awareness you gain, the more responsibility you gain. As you move through the various stages of awareness and awakening, you will see that life is about being comfortable with contrast. With knowing your pain and letting it go. With understanding your family and having compassion for them. For breaking the cycle of suffering. I knew from six years old that I was responsible for ending the cycle in my family. I knew I had to change the way my family saw their health and their bodies and how they lived their lives. But it was very hard for me to take the first step, to take some time out for myself and spend time in nature so I could listen to God. A lot of people couldn't understand it, but that was okay with me. A lot of people may not understand your journey, especially the people you are closest to, but that's okay. When you start changing, the people you are closest to will feel like they need to change, and that can be scary for them. Some may join you and kick-start their own journeys; others may decline and stay behind, comfortable in their current situation.

Your life will be determined by the people you surround yourself with because you usually share similar values, similar mindsets, and similar views of life. So the quickest way to change your life is by changing the people in it. It's true! If you want to get more out of life, if you want to move in a different direction, you must put yourself in places where people live the way you want to live. Sometimes that means walking away from family, from people who try to resist your change. You can still have compassion and patience for them without sabotaging your own growth and healing. If they want to grow with you, they will let you know. You have already started surrounding yourself with the right people by reading this book, by integrating these lessons and this energy into your mind, body, and soul. Only you can unlock your wildest dreams, those placed by God for you to fulfill and lean into, so that you can live your gifts out loud and invite the people around you to do the same, even if only by living in your truth.

Partnership

This journey of self-love often leads to finding your purpose partner and sharing a divine love that enhances and supports your mission, your goals, and what you want to accomplish in life. Sharing intimate love in a relationship is one of the most rewarding gifts you can receive from life. You can see yourself in each other. You can love each other through all the ups and downs, the highs and the lows. The dance between the masculine and the feminine energies, attracting your divine purpose partner, will help you to fulfill your dreams. The more you question your life and your relationships, the more your life and your relationships start to change. People will leave your life, and people will enter your life. This is the journey.

Relationships can be one of the most challenging aspects of the life journey because you are not only dealing with your own life and difficulties but you are also holding space for another human's life and difficulties. I learned very quickly on my journey that if I wanted to have fulfilling and meaningful relationships, I had to master the relationship with myself, express my most authentic self to the world, express my soul's essence, and allow myself to be seen for who I truly am. That was always the most challenging for me—to let myself be seen in all my different colors with all my amazing personalities because they're very contradictory at times! I always had a feeling that

I'm too much, that other people don't understand me, that I have to dim my light because I'm too loud or expressive. But what happened along my journey was that when I really and truly accepted myself, all of me not just part of me, when I became okay with the light aspects and the shadow aspects, I, ultimately, also honored all aspects of life.

You are already an expression of the whole. When you deny parts of yourself, you also deny certain aspects of life. Claiming back this power is one of the most magical things you can do for yourself. Once you reclaim the abandoned parts of yourself … once you integrate them into your being … you become focused and the path becomes clear. You experience a new sense of freedom and a deeper level of peace within yourself when you stop fighting against *you*. Theoretically, *knowing* your worth is great is only step one. *Embodying* the person that you truly love right here in this very moment is the real key. You are not here to hold yourself back or to live for "someday in the future." You are here to live all of life in the now. Beware of telling yourself, "I'll be more equipped or prepared when I have XYZ." In reality, you can always choose to be that person today.

Remember, thoughts are energetic. The more you tell yourself that the ideal version of you already exists, the easier it is to be that person. Plus, you'll be more likely to attract a partner that is compatible with that version. Stop the fight against yourself, the fight that says you aren't good enough or worthy of love, that you have to work hard to find love. Love won't come through a frequency of resistance; that is counterproductive. Stop fighting; instead, listen to your inner voice, your most authentic self, because this frequency will attract love.

What does your ideal partnership look like? What needs to happen so that you can feel the most free in society? In some aspects, your partner will complete you. But you also need to learn how to take responsibility for your emotions. Magic in a partnership happens when *you* take ownership for *your* life and *yourself* and really learn to deal with your internal reality and emotions exclusive of your partner. Like food, drugs, and alcohol, relationships, too, can be used to distract yourself from the way you feel inside. You may think these things make you happy, but it is always temporary, and eventually you have to face yourself again. There are no quick fixes in life; doing the uncomfortable work is the only way to lasting peace and happiness. If you are not able to be content with who you are when you are on your own, you will never be content in a relationship because true happiness cannot rely on external circumstances that can change at any moment. You cannot place your happiness in impermanence; the only thing you can truly control is what goes on inside you.

While it is beautiful to experience life with and through the eyes of another, it is just as beautiful to learn how to share that love with yourself; to learn how to nourish yourself and feed your mind, body, and soul in ways that make you feel alive.

This self-nourishment can help you counter loneliness. There are times in your life when you are in a dark space, a dark night of the soul, and it feels as though you are drowning; it feels as though you are sitting at the edge of a void. While this place can be very scary, it is also one of the most powerful experiences for growth of the human soul. Life is made up of both light and dark; you are ultimately alone in this human world, but awareness of this loneliness actually connects you to the source of all creation. When you understand that you are always connected to the Creator, you are never lost, you are never alone. It is only at the edge of the abyss that most people can understand this. It is during the darkest times of your life that the light of God can shine the brightest. This higher force will always lead you home, will always strengthen you and bring you back to peace. Home is within you. When you start to see that the cage around you is self-created, and that you can turn this cage into a safe nest, you realize that you don't need another person to feel complete.

Beauty can be born in periods of darkness and in void spaces, so it doesn't matter where you are on your journey right now. This is a process, and there is no wrong way to grow. When you said "yes" to this journey, you said "yes" to self-love, and self-love is about opening your heart to everything that is meant for you in this life. You said "yes" to opening yourself up to true connection, which is a journey for the brave. The brave ones, like you, don't shy away when it gets messy; you know deep down that you are connected to an amazing stream of love. You know how to ride these waves, to allow life to flow, to take life on. You are able to do great things by yourself, but beauty comes when you get to know the power of community and combining forces for good because this is true harmony: living in peace with yourself and peace with the world around you. When this happens, you can finally let go of toxic behaviors like hunting for a partner and staying in relationships because you are afraid of being alone, of supporting yourself financially, or because you don't know any better.

If you are willing to let go of these fears, willing to live from a place of wholeness, you will find the power within yourself to unleash the magic that you hold. You will set your soul free and open the door for true love, for healthy love, for relationships that are divine.

Try this ritual with yourself or with your partner. I actually recommend doing this by yourself first because it is a manifestation tool to call in your partner and to connect your souls. Find a sacred space in your home that makes you feel good. Play a song that feels sensual, sexual even, that lights a fire within you. Light a candle or sage, whatever makes you feel comfortable. Place some blankets and pillows on the ground and make a nest, a place for a sacred love meeting. Notice that in this sacred setting your whole being and body is more likely to open up to your feelings. Wear clothes that make you feel sexy or a fabric that your body enjoys. Sit in a comfortable position (and look at each other if you practice this with a partner), bringing your awareness to your body. Feel the ground beneath you; feel the fabric on your skin. Tell your body that it's safe—safe to get out of your mind and into your heart. Put your attention on your heart center; maybe feel it beating. Notice the energy coming from inside your heart center and radiating out to the world around you (or the person in front of you). Tune in to your senses. What can you hear, smell, taste, feel, and see?

If you're with a partner, open your eyes and look at them. Hold each other's hands. Look them in the eyes and be curious about what is in their universe. Whatever thoughts come up, just observe them like clouds and let them go. It's okay if you feel tears running down your face. When you feel like it's over, thank yourself or your partner for the experience and the vulnerability. You can repeat this exercise whenever you want, and include food like chocolate into the ritual if that is something that makes you feel good!

Another way to connect with your partner is to understand their love language. A love language is the way you receive and show love. There are five different love languages: gifts, acts of service, words of affirmation, quality time, and physical touch. It's important to know how you like to receive love, as well as how your partners, family, and friends receive love. Many women feel that they have to drag their partners on this journey because their partners aren't interested in discussing things like love languages. If this sounds like your relationship at the moment, focus on doing these intimate exercises with yourself and confronting any insecurities you feel about being intimate with *you*.

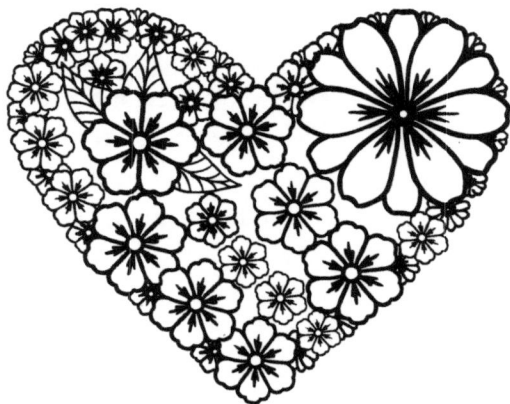

Purpose and the Divine

Learning how to connect with yourself and your community from a place of authenticity is how humanity starts to solve the problems of the world. Sickness comes from being misaligned with true purpose and the divine. When you live from a place of authenticity, you live from a place of love, and love is always pure. This is how you create heaven on Earth. Maybe you don't feel like a spiritual person; maybe you only picked this book up because you wanted to learn how to love yourself. Maybe you think that spirituality is nonsense and has nothing to do with life and reality and loving yourself. Maybe you think you aren't ready for spirituality, but I believe that human beings are born spiritual. I believe you are already spiritual, whether or not you are conscious of it. The more you embody your highest self, the more you embody God, the purest form of source energy. From this place, you will live in abundance—abundance for yourself and your life. Redefining spirituality and a spiritual connection is key to discovering your purpose.

You always have access to a higher source, and you can communicate with it for guidance. It knows the way. Even when you are stuck and it seems as though there is no way out, you can connect to the divine for answers. Living a life of purpose will lead you to places where you can't solve the problems with your logical mind.

Many life changes happen in divine timing. You must practice the virtues of patience, kindness, and compassion toward yourself because it helps you to be present for the messages and experiences that you receive from the divine. The Creator is so powerful that if you lean in and find a way, even without religious dogma, to connect to Him, you will become unstoppable. It's not about hustling; it's about asking yourself what kind of man or woman you want to be, and then allowing the process to unfold. This is the next step in your evolution. When you access that connection to the Creator, you will access the power to use your gifts for the greatest good.

Your connection with the divine will allow you to feel strong and confident. You will have improved health. You won't lack direction in life because you will have a clear mindset and life will appear rich and full of experiences that are here for you to live out loud. Remember, God placed these desires in your heart so that you can use them to experience the fullness of this life and who you are. God doesn't want to control you or force you; He longs for you to become aware of His presence, to become aware of the purpose you have been created for, and to be a vessel of love in this world. The spiritual journey is a journey of receiving—receiving love, receiving guidance, receiving peace.

Every morning, I devote myself to quiet time to receive from God. I become present and declare His loving presence over my life. One morning, as I said "I declare the loving presence of God over my life," a bird took flight and came to sit next to me. "Wow," I thought, "It's all true. This is the magic." When you believe and walk in faith, magic happens.

Your next step on the journey will always be revealed by your higher source in divine timing. It is always up to you to say "yes" when the next opportunity arises. Some opportunities appear subtly and without much warning; there will suddenly be a door or a person or a place that you are drawn to. Your soul will want you to say "yes" to this opportunity. You always have a choice to step fully through the door, to take a leap and not let your mind get in the way. Your mind will try to find reasons why you can't step through the door, why you shouldn't go to the place, why you can't say "yes" to that person. Your mind will tell you that you can't afford it, that there's not enough time, that you should do it later. And when you start observing these processes, you learn very quickly that all these opportunities are presented by God for you. So you can take the chance and shift your life and enjoy the life that you are meant to live. You are here to live in peace and harmony within yourself and with others.

A wonderful way to improve harmony with yourself and others is to focus on your routines. The power of routines is well-documented, but I see them as part of your journey toward purpose because routines become rituals.

There will come a time when all the walls around you that have been holding your illusion together collapse and you will be able to understand why you are here. You will finally understand your talents, your unique gifts, and how you can be a force for good in the world. Recognizing your own magnificence, your own beauty, your own power, you will see that you are the one you have been waiting for. Starting your day with a morning ritual frames your mind for the day and sets its trajectory so that you can continue to live in alignment with these revelations of your magnificence and power. Rituals anchor you in who you are; they ground you to the awareness of your life. They act as a remembrance of everything you are fighting for and everything you are becoming. I love taking walks in the morning to ground myself, to speak to my soul, to stretch my body and mind, and to remember how amazing the Creator is and how amazing I am as a creation.

Start your day with a ritual, and allow yourself to be a vessel for the bounty and beauty of life, to let the love of life flow through you. It is from this place that all relationships start.

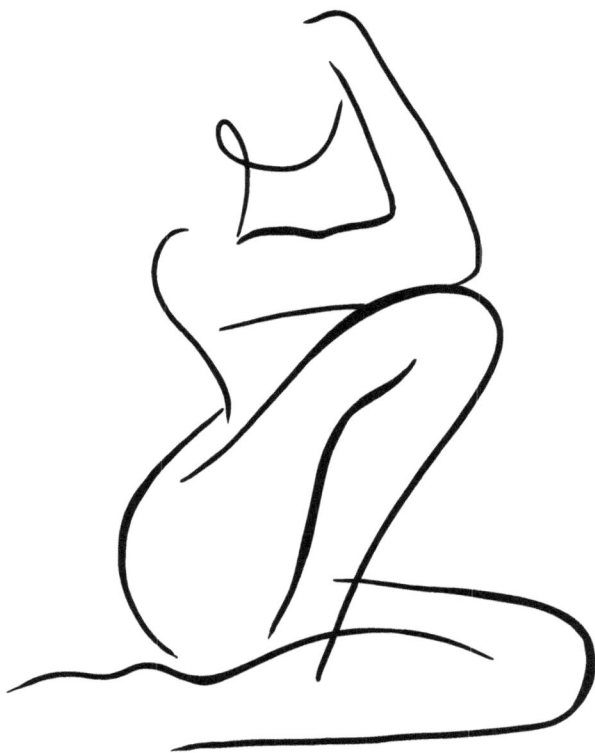

CHAPTER 6
EASE & GRACE

Accept

Now that you know how life is supposed to feel and understand that you have been created for a purpose and a relationship with the Creator, you can start to live from a place of alignment and ease. You know now that you can't experience love when you start from a place of judgment and hate. But, of course, this is easier said than done.

Look at the following Hawkins scale of emotions. As you can see, human beings have different emotions, and each emotion has a different frequency. The goal of this journey is to create a life that feels good on the inside. You want to radiate light from the inside out. I have been through a lot of valleys and dark times in my life, times when I didn't know whether I would make it to the next day. I started my journey because I felt emotionally disconnected from life, and I needed a shift. But starting from a place of feeling not good enough could not attract the abundance and happiness I sought. Operating from lower frequency emotions won't attract higher frequency emotions. You cannot create abundance from scarcity. In order to achieve the fullness of life, you must accept that all these emotions, all these frequencies, exist. There is energy all around you.

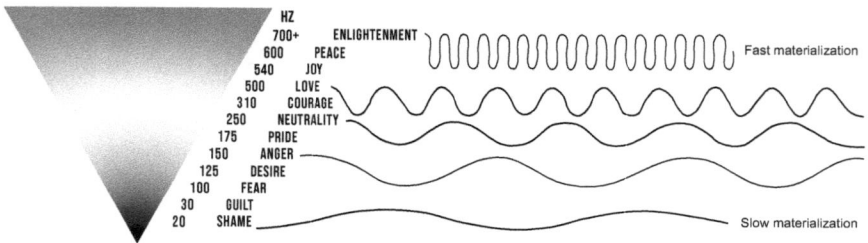

HZ
700+ ENLIGHTENMENT
600 PEACE
540 JOY
500 LOVE
310 COURAGE
250 NEUTRALITY
175 PRIDE
150 ANGER
125 DESIRE
100 FEAR
30 GUILT
20 SHAME

Fast materialization

Slow materialization

I had to start with acceptance. I had to accept how I felt about myself. I had to accept that life wasn't always going to be joyful and peaceful and that I had to take the good with the bad. When you choose to open yourself up to life, you choose to be open to *all* of life. If you can't accept the place you are now, you cannot move beyond that place. I had to accept my health and my reality as it looked in that moment. Acceptance is neutrality. It is seeing things as they are and not as you want them to be. There is no resistance. Becoming honest about the way your life looks right now, and then making peace with that reality, is how you move in a new direction. You can experience all your emotions in that moment without becoming attached to them—without making the emotions your identity. It is an experience of your reality, not reality itself.

Ask yourself who you would be without the shame and guilt. What would you do differently if you weren't attached to those emotions? The more you resist those emotions, the more you constrict their flow through your body. This is how you become sick and resentful. Once you can accept your reality and how you feel about it, you will allow the emotions to flow. Processing emotions in this way is how you make the shift in your life. On one side, you have to accept that all emotions exist, and, on the other side, you have to accept that there is also love waiting to flow through you.

I realized on my own journey that as soon as I was truly ready to put all of this awareness into practice, as soon as I said, "Yes, I am ready," I implemented Chapter 1 in my life. Then I did everything in Chapter 2 and experienced my life through my senses. Then I learned everything I could about my energy and started creating. And when I started shifting thoughts and beliefs and, thus, my identity, my outer realities started shifting, and, suddenly, I noticed that everything was working for my good. The inner work created outward shifts. I looked at my life from a new perspective, from a neutral place of acceptance rather than through the eyes of a victim. I started appreciating everything that had happened to me that had brought me to that moment, to being that person.

But when I started feeling joy, I simultaneously felt resistance to the joy because my lifestyle was changing. Though I was getting everything I sought, I could feel old parts of me wanting to go back to the way things had been before. So I realized I had to prepare myself and my body for this joy, for the abundance that was flowing in. I allowed myself to experience the reality of all my emotions, acknowledging the fear before letting go of it.

I was so used to experiencing intense, low frequency emotions that made my body sick, that I had to increase the capacity for blissful emotions. I had to learn to hold love in my body. I had to learn to accept every emotion, all the energy that wanted to flow. I had to learn to receive with ease, to allow things to be as they were. When you grow up watching everyone around you struggle, fighting for love, for money, for attention, for survival, it is a whole new experience to suddenly get everything you want and need. I had to change the lens through which I was observing life, rewiring my brain to see new things that were different from the old patterns. Through the lens of divine love, I was able to finally experience abundance and pure love.

When I visited Los Angeles, I went to the Hollywood Walk of Fame. The city was bustling with people taking photographs, people who appeared to be happy and have everything they needed. Ten minutes down the road, that same city was full of unhoused people. Life is duality; life is contrast. It's important to never forget this, to never forget that life is full of abundance but also extreme suffering. Try to put yourself in situations where you can be open to life to see the contrast—to experience the duality. You need to live from a place of understanding all emotions, not running and escaping the uncomfortable ones, so that you can embody all of your humanity and use all of your gifts for the greater good, to change the world, change the cities, change the lives of your fellow human beings. When I travel to cities I have already visited, I like to see the way things are evolving, to see the ways I am evolving as a person, to see how my mindset shifts. I think back on how I previously perceived the very same place and understand how much I have grown since then. I am able to see the work of God in my life in these moments, to entrust my life to the Creator, and to ask Him what comes next because I have made it this far, and I am still moving forward. I have made it this far yet there is still so much for me to do to change the world. I want to leave a legacy of love, to create something that will last long after I have left this planet.

This must start from a place of acceptance because acceptance is where love flows. This is who you truly are. This is worth writing down in your journal and thinking about over the next few days. You have the choice to be a blessing in this life to yourself and to other people, to show up in a way that serves humanity with your gifts and your love. Acceptance is the first step in this journey followed by allowing, releasing, and then receiving. This is enlightenment. You are here to have it all, and a life lived this way is a life of ease. Your soul knows the way. So make a plan. Move into action to fulfill that plan, taking care of yourself every step of the way so that you can accomplish what you have been created for.

Allow

Most people live their lives waiting for permission from others to have everything they want to have and to do everything they want to do. But true alignment comes when you are able to give yourself permission, to allow yourself to be the way you want to be, and to live your life the way you want to live it. This is the gift you give yourself: permission to have it all. This is how you allow blessings and emotions to flow. You are the fullest expression of God and all creation when you are living all of life, all experiences—light and dark.

Take a look at yourself in the mirror. When you look into your eyes, you are looking into the universe. When you talk out loud to yourself, you are talking to God and to the universe and all of creation that lives inside you. See who you are, and allow yourself to be the fullness of who you have been created to be. Now, speak out loud to your reflection and to God what you want to allow into your life. When you *accept* yourself and your circumstances as they are in this moment, when you *allow* yourself and your circumstances to be as they are in this moment, you have your power back in your hands. You can choose to make a new plan for your life. It's important your focus is not on what you need to take away because restricting and depriving yourself drains your energy. Shift your attention to *more*.

- What feels amazing?
- What do you need more of?
- What blessing can you allow into your life?

Go toward what fills your cup; go toward the frequency of abundance. This mirror work is one of the most powerful tools that you can use to practice choosing abundance. The key is to not speak something to the mirror that you don't believe is for you; meet yourself where you are at and start from there.

When I talk to myself in the mirror, I allow myself to feel my energy in that moment and hold myself in a place of joy. I look myself in the eyes, and I know I'm a good person. I know I am beautiful. I even enjoy eating chocolate in front of the mirror. I know where I come from. I remember the times I stood in front of the mirror hating my body, hating myself, talking negatively about who I was. And seeing myself as I am now, able to feel and know love for myself, makes me fall in love with myself even more. And because I did it, I know you can, too. I never gave up on the love for myself. I never gave up on myself, and I never stopped believing in myself. I always stood up and found a new way and a different solution. And in times when I didn't know what to do next, I asked my Creator for help and allowed myself to connect with the intimacy of life again.

And I just kept repeating this practice. Even when I didn't see results on the outside, I knew deep down that I loved myself, and I would never stop loving myself until it was done. This is a commitment you can make to yourself to show yourself how worthy, how magnificent you are. You can use everything in this world to either dim your light or to enhance your relationship with yourself. And you get to decide which path you choose. You have the power. Even if nobody believes in you, even if nobody understands it, this is your commitment to yourself, and nothing can stop you from honoring it. It is using self-love practices to actually love yourself. It is using food as a tool for playfulness to make your light shine and to light up the world. For more self-love practices, visit **carolineickhoff.com/free**.

The secret to healing a broken relationship with food is to heal the relationship with yourself. It is committing to radical

THE SECRET OF FOOD

self-inquiry on a quest to love yourself. When you learn to move and eat and talk in a way that honors your body and soul, you achieve unlimited potential for growth and change. It is from this place that your relationship with health, with money, and with love will flourish. This book isn't a challenge; it isn't something you do for a few weeks. It is an invitation to actively participate in your evolution. It is a commitment to honor your heart and your life. It is a commitment to pay attention to your body, mind, and soul and give yourself permission to move and act with purpose.

Release

Releasing is always about control. Understanding that you have a need to control because you are looking for certainty and safety allows you to understand why it can be so difficult to release what you are still holding on to. Surrendering to this process is about trusting yourself and God enough to know that you don't need to hold the whole universe together. That you can release your grip and allow love to flow through you. One of the best ways to allow release is to move your body. You can't intellectualize release; it must be moved through action, through the movement of energy. You can't think the weight away. You need to move the stuck energy out of your system so that you can operate from a different frequency. Once you have learned to release control, it won't come back because there is no need for it.

You can release all kinds of things in addition to control—people, places, circumstances, things that you thought you knew, things that you thought you needed. Check to see if you're holding onto things that make you feel stuck and stagnant within yourself. Raise your hand in a fist in front of you, and squeeze very hard. Put all your attention on your fist, and try to imagine the things you are holding onto. Notice how it feels in your body trying to hold your fist. Now, let go and open your hand. Feel the release. Feel the grace of letting go and opening up. This is how it is to release emotions, to let go of what you are holding onto, to move with grace from closed to open. Feel the freedom in the release. Now, you can fly. Your soul can breathe. Your heart is open. There is a shift inside you; you are light.

You can also release shame from this place. Shame is one of the lowest frequency emotions, and releasing it allows you to shift your mindset from "I am worthless" to "I am doing my best, I am learning, I am practicing. I am allowed to experience love." This is your evolution; this is you breaking free from your self-imprisonment. You are releasing so that you are free to create the life you desire.

Receive

Once you have released, you are ready to receive. Focus on what you want to release and what you want to receive in its place. Focus on yourself—not your kids, not your family, not your friends—focus on what *you* want to receive. Maybe you notice that it's easier for you to receive for others than it is to receive for yourself. But notice what it is you want to receive, and be willing to receive it. Be open to the miracles that come when you start to release, when you become vulnerable and ask for what you need. Miracles can become normal in your life. They don't happen when you try to control them, when you try to make them happen on your terms. When you release control, you are connected to the source and everything that is available to you becomes possible, even things you didn't know existed. This is the fun part. As soon as you are ready to receive, as soon as you focus your mind on what you want and need to accomplish your purpose, you will start to gain clarity about your path, and the universe can work in your favor. The universe can align everything around you to present the opportunities and possibilities to you. God wants to give this all to you. God wants you so badly to fall in love with this way of living, to receive the abundance and all the gifts that are waiting for you. It is amazing what happens when you say "yes" over and over again to the possibilities that are all around you.

It is possible, and the minute you decide it's possible, it's already done. God is doing miraculous things with your life. God is speaking to you through people, places, circumstances, animals, and nature; you only have to be a little bit open and flexible to receive and to hear His voice.

Food was always a way for me to numb and distract myself or to regulate my intense emotions. But if you learn how to feel these emotions, to release what you can't control, to stop suppressing them, you can use food to navigate through life. Whenever I missed the sweetness of life, whenever I had the feeling that I wasn't fully living, I used food to satisfy the craving for sweetness, as well as the love I was missing. The moment I realized that I am the love and that it comes from the inside out, I could feed my whole being in a new way. I started receiving love from the sun, allowing the tingling sensations of sunlight on my skin to nourish me. Energetic foods came into my life, and I noticed that when I spent more time with people and in places I truly loved, I was less hungry. I started slowing down and listening to the divine, allowing myself to be in the present moment, connecting with my senses and enhancing the awareness that came with them. I was able to be more open and receptive to life, to receiving blessings. I spoke more gently to myself. Instead of soothing my emotions with food, I allowed myself to have my emotions and practiced loving myself from this space.

And then I had peace within me because I realized I was ready for my next chapter, the next level of what it felt like to be the love of my own life. I felt grounded and present. And it all started with two questions: "What would my life look like if I truly loved myself? How would life look if I was willing to accept the answers I got?" Because after you receive it, you must act. You must put it into your schedule, make it real, be willing to try and fail. There isn't ever really failure when you are on a journey toward loving yourself. You are already the love you are seeking. There is no place to get to because you are already there; there is nothing to accomplish because you are already it.

CHAPTER 7
TRUTH & TRUST

Discernment

In the journey of life, there are many paths to choose from, each presenting its own set of opportunities and challenges. Amidst myriad choices, discernment emerges as a guiding light, offering clarity, wisdom, and insight to navigate the twists and turns of your existence. But what exactly is discernment, and how can you cultivate this quality in your life so that you can become a vessel for divine guidance and purpose?

Discernment is more than just making decisions; it's about tapping into your inner wisdom and spiritual intuition to ascertain what is true, just, and aligned with your highest good. It involves the ability to perceive and understand the deeper meaning behind people, situations, and information, allowing you to make choices that are in alignment with your values, purpose, and spiritual path.

Discernment permeates every aspect of your life, from the relationships you cultivate to the decisions you make and the paths you choose to follow. It empowers you to distinguish between truth and falsehood, light and darkness, love and fear, guiding you toward greater authenticity, integrity, and alignment with your divine purpose.

As vessels for God's wisdom and love, it is imperative that you cultivate the gift of discernment in your life. By honing your spiritual intuition and deepening your connection with the divine, you will become attuned to the subtle whispers of the Holy Spirit guiding you along the path of righteousness and divine alignment. Love serves as a potent catalyst for the development of discernment. When you approach life with an open heart and a spirit of love and compassion, you create space for divine wisdom to flow freely into your life. Love enables you to see beyond surface appearances, connecting you with the essence of people and situations and guiding you toward decisions that are rooted in kindness, empathy, and divine love.

Food, too, can play a role in learning discernment. By cultivating mindful eating practices and honoring the sacredness of food, you deepen your connection with the divine source of nourishment that sustains you. As you savor each bite with gratitude and reverence, you attune your senses to the subtle energies of the universe, heightening your awareness and intuition and fostering a deeper understanding of your body's needs and the interconnectedness of all life.

By cultivating discernment in your life, you become a vessel for God's love and wisdom, channeling divine guidance and purpose into every aspect of your existence. So embrace the gift of discernment, trusting in the divine wisdom that dwells within you and allowing love and nourishment to support you on your journey toward spiritual growth, fulfillment, and divine alignment.

Love Is the Answer

What a beautiful ride. I'm smiling because I know where you started in the book, and I know how much your life will blossom when you put these principles into action and create the life that you have always dreamed of. Truth is the key to your vision, to an abundance of energy, to being one with everything around you and feeling whole. You are coming back to the feelings you have uncovered on this journey. But do you actually trust that you are love, that you are already the answer to your own life? Can you use your discernment to determine if this is all true for you?

I want you to have a look at what you believe is true for you. It's all that matters. I had to learn how to discern again and again. Consider that everything you want is a buffet. Take your golden platter and put everything you want to experience and everything you want to receive on it. Now, understand that not everything on the platter is truth; it becomes true when you decide that it is true for you. You have to learn how to take what is true for you, how to choose what you want, and how to leave what you don't want.

You must learn to master the truth for yourself. You must learn to stop listening to all the voices and people telling you what is true, and tune into your own heart and body. Ask yourself, "Does this feel true for me? What is my truth? What do I want to believe?" It's easy to become sidetracked by teachers, trainers, and people you admire. But it's time to take those people off their pedestals. Nobody goes in front of you, nobody goes behind you, nobody goes beneath you or above you. You are connected to all things, and you can honor yourself and your truth and know that it is enough. Listen to your own intuition and guidance, know that it is truth, and rely on it.

You have likely heard a lot about listening to your intuition or inner voice. God's voice is a whisper. It is soft and loving, not loud and obnoxious. That is society's voice. Other people's opinions sound like: "You should, you must." The way you identify God's voice, intuition, from the noise is by listening for the stillness, the quiet, the whisper. It sounds like, "Yes. It's for you. Do this." It feels loving and supportive and never fails. It will always guide you to beauty and goodness. You can live by this truth. So ask yourself, "What is my truth?" And learn to listen for and trust the answer that comes in the whisper. Trust in the self-love journey is very important because you need to be able to trust that if you say you are committing to yourself, you are.

Waterfalls

This is the moment when you have to practice saying something and then doing it. This is trust. Not saying "yes" but meaning "no." Too often, that is the pattern for people who are sick and overweight. They are so busy doing things for other people, busy putting everyone else first and hiding their own needs, that they end up last in their own lives. This needs to change—radically, right now. You need to say "yes" to what you mean ... to what you want ... and actually follow up and do it.

Establishing trust with yourself means you can count on yourself, that you know you will look after yourself and your needs. This helps you build self-worth and trust the wisdom that comes from within. Telling yourself you are going to do something and actually following through is one of the ways you show yourself that you deserve love and good things! Your body needs this kind of trust, too. I teach people how to transform in a sustainable way because most people's bodies don't believe they are capable of change anymore because they are constantly stepping on their own boundaries and acting in ways that aren't good for them. On my journey, I not only had to become friends with myself and my body again, but I also needed to trust God and life again. When I started doing that, life started trusting me. I strengthened my ability to say out loud, "Thank you for this gift." And now I'm doing it and following through with what I said.

It is very beautiful when your body reflects that trust back. Your body is learning that you actually mean it and that you will never stop loving yourself again. There will be times when life is wild, and you will have to remember yourself again. But it is a journey that you can commit yourself to for your whole life because you are honoring and trusting yourself through the process. Your body is inhaling and exhaling energy, whether in the form of food, money, or experiences. It just flows. So step into the flow of life again.

I always picture a waterfall in the beautiful jungle of Costa Rica when I think of flow. I remember the exact moment I stood in a beautiful national park after having hiked for two hours to find the purest water on Earth. It was refreshing to be in such an energetic place. I took off my clothes and lowered myself into the water when, suddenly, the waterfall started talking to me. The presence of God was, once again, right there. When I tune in and I'm receptive to it, I experience life in a profoundly ethereal way.

The waterfall said to me, "Come closer, come closer." I started laughing. I thought, "Okay, I will come closer and closer to you." I looked up, right to the top, and saw a glorious rainbow shining its beautiful colors over the whole jungle, and I was in awe. That had always been my sign, the rainbow. It had always been my anchor, a signal that I was on track. I felt pure bliss and joy underneath that waterfall, thanking God and thinking, "Does it get any better than this? Thank you. I thank you from the bottom of my heart for playing with me and showing me how beautiful life is, how amazing love feels, how magical nature can be."

The waterfall kept talking to me. I know that you're laughing again, but maybe you've had an experience like this somewhere, somehow. God is constantly using your external reality to talk to you. I was so close to His voice that day, and He asked me to open my arms, and I said, "Okay, I am here." I opened them wide. He then asked me to go under the waterfall and just stand in the stream of flowing water. I stepped into it, and I cried from the bottom of my lungs. I couldn't breathe. I felt so blessed, reaching for the stars in the waterfall, remembering the rainbow right above me, and I suddenly got it. I had arrived. God is here because I am here.

In that moment, I understood that God was using me as a vessel to express this love that life has for everyone. I knew that this was true, this feeling of being that is divine purpose. I watched the water flow and realized that this was abundance—a never-ending flow. It never stops. And I realized that I could choose to step to the side, to step out of the flow, or I could choose to stay submerged in the flow. It was my choice to step in and out of the stream of life. The minute I moved to the right or to the left, I was no longer in the stream. The moment you open your arms and your heart, you are letting divine presence flow through and to you; you are part of abundance and love. You, too, are the expression of and source of this higher power.

So it is true that you can choose to tune in to this experience; it is a radio dial. You can tune yourself to the perfect frequency, to the perfect vibration, and you can enhance this vibration by loving yourself, taking care of yourself, feeding yourself, and calibrating yourself using energetic foods. You can use all of the tools in this book to tune your energy to the stream of life. So ask yourself, "Where am I standing?" Use your senses to see, smell, taste, hear, and touch the waterfall. Use hydration and nutrition, good sleep, movement, and self-care to prepare your body to stand in the stream of light and flow and love. Think it, believe it, take action. Now, you can celebrate yourself beneath the magnificent waterfall. Yes, you are here. You are one with the divine. You have established a connection where you can accept, allow, release, and receive the abundance. You have decided that *this* is your truth. You now know that you can trust yourself and that you were the secret all along.

LOVE BALL

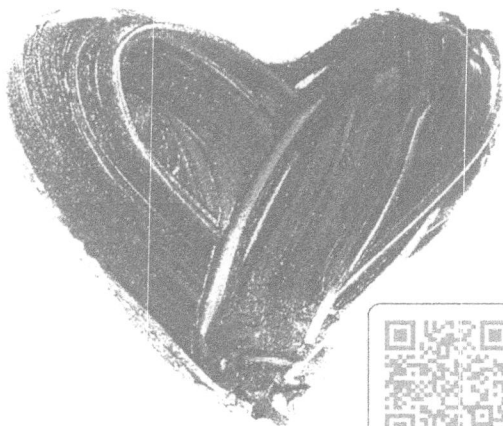

LOVE FOOD
RECIPES

Peanut Butter Banana Protein Smoothie

INGREDIENTS:

1 ripe banana

1 tablespoon natural
  peanut butter

½ cup almond milk
  (or any plant-based milk
  of your choice)

¼ cup rolled oats

1 scoop of vegan protein powder
  (vanilla or chocolate flavored)

INSTRUCTIONS:

- Peel the banana and break it into chunks.
- In a blender, add the banana chunks, peanut butter, almond milk, rolled oats, and vegan protein powder.
- Blend until smooth and creamy. If the smoothie is too thick, add a little more almond milk until you reach your desired consistency.
- Pour into a glass and enjoy immediately!

PRAYER:

"Dear God, thank you for providing us with nourishing foods to fuel our bodies. May this smoothie remind us of your love and care for our well-being, and may it strengthen us to fulfill your purpose for our lives. Amen."

Berry Blast Protein Smoothie

INGREDIENTS:

½ cup frozen mixed berries (strawberries, blueberries, raspberries)

½ cup silken tofu (soft tofu)

½ cup spinach leaves (fresh or frozen)

1 tablespoon chia seeds

½ cup coconut water (or plain water)

INSTRUCTIONS:

- In a blender, combine the frozen mixed berries, silken tofu, spinach leaves, chia seeds, and coconut water.
- Blend until everything is smooth and well combined. If the smoothie is too thick, add a little more coconut water until you reach your desired consistency.
- Taste the smoothie and adjust sweetness if necessary by adding a drizzle of maple syrup or a few drops of liquid stevia.
- Pour into a glass and enjoy the burst of berry flavor!

PRAYER:

"Dear God, thank you for the abundance of fruits and vegetables that nourish our bodies. As we enjoy this vibrant smoothie, may it fill us with your goodness and grant us the strength to serve you joyfully each day. Amen."

Green Goddess Power Smoothie

INGREDIENTS:

1 ripe banana

1 cup fresh spinach leaves

½ ripe avocado

½ cup frozen pineapple chunks

1 tablespoon hemp seeds

½ cup coconut water

(or plain water)

INSTRUCTIONS:

- Peel the banana and break it into chunks.
- Cut the avocado in half, remove the pit, and scoop out the flesh.
- In a blender, combine the banana chunks, fresh spinach leaves, avocado flesh, frozen pineapple chunks, hemp seeds, and coconut water.
- Blend until smooth and creamy. If the smoothie is too thick, add a little more coconut water until you reach your desired consistency.
- Taste the smoothie and adjust sweetness if necessary by adding a drizzle of maple syrup or a few drops of liquid stevia.
- Pour into a glass and enjoy the green goodness!

PRAYER:

"Gracious God, thank you for the gift of health and vitality. As we partake in this nourishing green smoothie, may it fill us with your strength and renew our bodies and minds. May your greatness be reflected in our actions as we strive to glorify you in all we do. Amen."

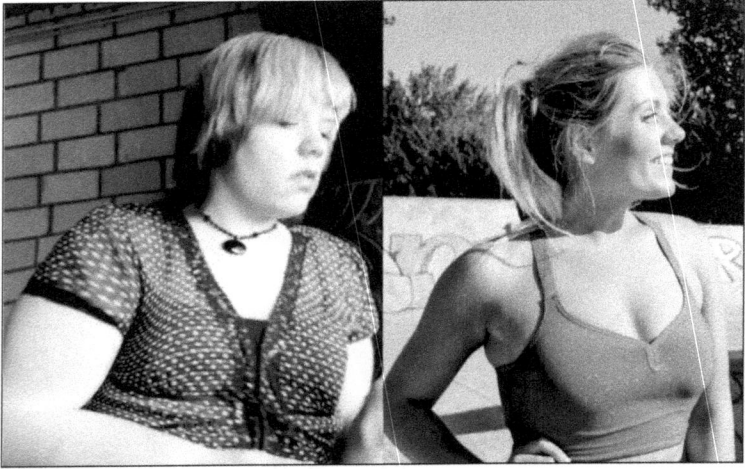

To connect with Carolin and
learn more about her work, visit

carolineickhoff.com

@carolineickhoff

ABOUT THE AUTHOR

Carolin Eickhoff's life story is a testament to resilience and transformation. From grappling with obesity and health issues, she embarked on a remarkable journey that saw her shed 130 pounds and reclaim her vitality and power. As the visionary founder of the Love Ball and the My Best Version Academy for sustainable nutrition, and the host of the My Best Version podcast, Carolin has become an internationally recognized figure in the wellness sphere. Her international best-selling book, *The Secret of Food: Divine Nourishment for Self-Love and Radiant Health*, encapsulates her journey, offering readers a roadmap to holistic healing and self-discovery. With her unique blend of depth, humor, and kindness, Carolin inspires millions to embrace their bodies, love themselves, and live a life filled with joy and nourishment.

Her impact extends beyond her book and academy; through her non-profit organization, a food for purpose initiative, she is saving lives by providing nutritious meals to communities in need worldwide, helping children build a better future by leading them toward a life of abundance and possibility.

Carolin's approach to wellness emphasizes sustainable practices and a deep connection to food as a source of nourishment for both body and soul. With her infectious energy and unwavering commitment to making a difference, she continues to inspire individuals to embrace their true selves and live life to the fullest.

9 78 1 9 56 83 7 35 3